CLINICAL AND EXPERIMENTAL PSYCHIATRY

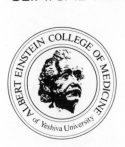

*Monograph Series
of the Department of Psychiatry
Albert Einstein College of Medicine/
Montefiore Medical Center
New York, N.Y.*

CLINICAL AND EXPERIMENTAL PSYCHIATRY
Monograph Series

Clinical and Experimental Psychiatry Monograph No. 2

COMPUTER APPLICATIONS IN PSYCHIATRY AND PSYCHOLOGY

Edited by

David Baskin, Ph.D.

Department of Psychiatry
Albert Einstein College of Medicine
of Yeshiva University/
Montefiore Medical Center
New York, N.Y.

BRUNNER/MAZEL Publishers • New York

Library of Congress Cataloging-in-Publication Data

Computer applications in psychiatry and psychology / edited by David
Baskin.
     p.   cm. — (Clinical and experimental psychiatry ; 2)
   Includes bibliographies and index.
   ISBN 0-87630-539-7
   1. Psychiatry—Data processing.   2. Psychology—Data processing.
3. Microcomputers.   I. Baskin, David.   II. Series.
   [DNLM: 1. Computers.   2. Psychiatry.   3. Psychology.   WM 26.5
C738]
   RC455.2.D38C66   1989
   616.89'00285—dc20
   DNLM/DLC
   for Library of Congress   89-17277
                                                                  CIP

Copyright © 1990 by Albert Einstein College
of Medicine of Yeshiva University

Published by
BRUNNER/MAZEL, INC.
19 Union Square
New York, New York 10003

MANUFACTURED IN THE UNITED STATES OF AMERICA

10 9 8 7 6 5 4 3 2 1

A NOTE ON THE SERIES

Psychiatry is in a state of flux. The excitement springs in part from internal changes, such as the development and official acceptance (at least in the U.S.A.) of an operationalized, multiaxial classification system of behavioral disorders (the DSM-III), the increasing sophistication of methods to measure abnormal human behavior and the impressive expansion of biological and psychological treatment modalities. Exciting developments are also taking place in fields relating to psychiatry; in molecular (brain) biology, genetics, brain imaging, drug development, epidemiology, experimental psychology, to mention only a few striking examples.

More generally speaking, psychiatry is moving, still relatively slowly, but irresistibly, from a more philosophical, contemplative orientation, to that of an empirical science. From the fifties on, biological psychiatry has been a major catalyst of that process. It provided the mother discipline with a third cornerstone, i.e., neurobiology, the other two being psychology and medical sociology. In addition, it forced the profession into the direction of standardization of diagnoses and of assessment of abnormal behavior. Biological psychiatry provided psychiatry not only with a new basic science and with new treatment modalities, but also with the tools, the methodology and the mentality to operate within the confines of an empirical science, the only framework in which a medical discipline can survive.

In other fields of psychiatry, too, one discerns a gradual trend towards scientification. Psychological treatment techniques are standardized and manuals developed to make these skills more easily transferable. Methods registering treatment outcome—traditionally used in the behavioral/cognitive field—are now more and more requested and, hence, developed for dynamic forms of psychotherapy as well. Social and community psychiatry, until the sixties more firmly rooted in humanitarian ideals and social awareness than in empirical studies, profited greatly from its liaison with the social sciences, and the expansion of psychiatric epidemiology.

Let there be no misunderstanding. Empiricism does *not imply* that it is only the measurable that counts. Psychiatry would be mutilated if it would neglect that what is not yet capturable in numbers and probably never will be. It *does imply* that what is measurable should be measured. Progress in psychiatry is dependent on ideas and on experiment. Their linkage is inseparable.

This monograph series, published under the auspices of the Department of Psychiatry of the Albert Einstein College of Medicine/Montefiore Medical Center, is meant to keep track of important developments in our profession, to summarize what has been achieved in particular fields, and to bring together the viewpoints obtained from disparate vantage points—in short, to capture some of the excitement ongoing in modern psychiatry, both in its clinical and experimental dimensions. Our Department hosts the Series, but naturally welcomes contributions from others.

Bernie Mazel is not only the publisher of this series, but it was he who generated the idea—an ambitious plan which, however, we all feel is worthy of pursuit. The edifice of psychiatry is impressive, but still somewhat flawed in its foundations. May this Series contribute to consolidation of its infrastructure.

HERMAN M. VAN PRAAG, M.D., PH.D.
Silverman Professor and Chairman
Albert Einstein College of Medicine/
Montefiore Medical Center
Department of Psychiatry
Bronx, New York   *U.S.A.*

CONTENTS

CONTRIBUTORS

David Baskin, Ph.D.
Associate Professor of Psychiatry, Albert Einstein College of Medicine; Associate Director, Sound View-Throgs Neck, Community Mental Health Center of Albert Einstein College of Medicine, New York, New York

Peter Ericson, B.A.
Director of Information Services, Institute of Living, Hartford, Connecticut

David Gastfriend, M.D.
Assistant Professor of Psychiatry, Harvard Medical School; Chief, West End Group Practice, Alcohol & Drug Treatment Unit; Director, Psychopharmacology Research & Clinical Information System, Massachusetts General Hospital, Boston, Massachusetts

John H. Greist, M.D.
Professor of Psychiatry, University of Wisconsin Medical School, Madison, Wisconsin

Toksoz B. Karasu, M.D.

Deputy Chairman and Professor of Psychiatry, Albert Einstein College of Medicine, New York, New York

Robert S. Kennedy, M.A.

Coordinator of Clinical Information Systems, Coordinator of Residency Training, Department of Psychiatry, Albert Einstein College of Medicine, New York, New York

Robert Plutchik, Ph.D.

Professor of Psychiatry, Albert Einstein College of Medicine, New York, New York

James Robinson, B.A.

Director, Information Sciences Division, The Nathan S. Kline Institute, Orangeburg, New York

Marc D. Schwartz, M.D.

Associate Research Professor of Psychiatry, New York University; Editor, *Computers in Psychiatry/Psychology,* New Haven, Connecticut

Samuel Seiffer, M.A.

Associate in Psychiatry, Albert Einstein College of Medicine; Director of Information Services, Sound View-Throgs Neck, Community Mental Health Center of Albert Einstein College of Medicine, New York, New York

Herman M. van Praag, M.D., Ph.D.

Chairman, Dept. of Psychiatry, Albert Einstein College of Medicine, New York, New York

Scott Wetzler, Ph.D.

Head, Clinical Assessment Program, Division of Psychology; Assistant Professor of Psychiatry, Albert Einstein College of Medicine, New York, New York

PREFACE

The burgeoning of the utilization of computers in the fields of psychiatry and psychology during the past ten years has had a significant impact on training, research and service within these fields.

This monograph includes material from a tristate symposium on Computer Applications in Psychiatry held at the Albert Einstein College of Medicine in New York City, as well as additional articles especially prepared for this publication.

In Part 1, Dr. Herman van Praag, Chairman of the Department of Psychiatry at Albert Einstein, and I offer a brief introduction and overview of the field.

Part 2 is dedicated to clinical applications of computers, especially psychiatric diagnosis. Dr. Marc Schwartz offers an overview of applications, including word processing, database programs and psychological testing. He also points out the ethical responsibility of the practitioner in using computers. Dr. John Greist comprehensively examines the use of computers in formulating psychiatric diagnosis.

He also proffers valuable insight into the psychological effects of computer use on practitioners and how an awareness of these effects may minimize resistance to utilization.

Drs. Robert Plutchik and Byram Karasu present a comprehensive review of the literature with regard to computers as interviewers, computers as psychotherapists and computers as patients. The authors also discuss the implications of the uses of computers. Dr. Scott Wetzler scrutinizes the use of computerized psychological assessment, with a critical evaluation of such use.

The third part presents two chapters that focus on the establishment of databases in mental health systems. The chapter by Robert Kennedy explains the rudiments of setting up databases for patient management in a mental health system. Accurate, timely, and complete patient records are essential to management, who have become increasingly accountable to regulating and funding agencies. Dr. Gastfriend explicates how computerized database files can be used in psychopharmacology for research and clinical care. Both of these chapters yield pragmatic recommendations for the novitiate as well as for the more sophisticated.

Part 4 is devoted to computerized management information systems. Jim Robinson discusses general uses and content of mental health information systems, types of patient and fiscal data, operational characteristics of such systems, and hardware considerations. Peter Ericson presents the real operation of a computerized information system, including networking and an actual sample of what a report actually looks like. Sam Seiffer also presents a practical example of how a computer, in this case a microcomputer, can be employed in a management information system for a continuing treatment psychiatric rehabilitation program.

The last part relates the findings of a nationwide survey of computer utilization in community mental health centers.

High technology and computers have been rapidly making their way into health care systems, and in particular into the mental health service delivery system. To date, no examination on a nationwide basis has been made as to how computers are being used in mental health. This study examines this issue.

A total of 648 community mental health centers were sent questionnaires requesting information with regard to characteristics of their respective centers and of their utilization of computers. Two hundred and fifty-six (256) centers responded, constituting a 40% response rate.

An important finding of the study was that even though computerization was not perceived to have reduced costs, it was perceived as having increased the efficiency of the organization.

The significance of this study is that it has chronicled the advent of widespread utilization of computers in community mental health centers.

ACKNOWLEDGMENT

The editor wishes to express his gratitude to Ms. Catherine Harnett for her transcribing and typing of the manuscript.

DAVID BASKIN, PH.D.

PART I

INTRODUCTION AND OVERVIEW

COMPUTERS IN PSYCHIATRY: A MISSED OPPORTUNITY

Herman M. van Praag

Imagine a department of psychiatry, responsible for mental health delivery in a borough of about 1.2 million people, of which approximately 5,000 per year are admitted to its psychiatric beds. Many patients, fortunately, are improved at discharge, but they are not cured. Many need aftercare; many will visit emergency rooms in the future; and for many, readmission will become inevitable in the forseeable future.

The number of visits to psychiatric clinics affiliated with that imaginary department is correspondingly high, approximately 600,000 per year, while 15,000 clients are yearly being seen in its emergency rooms. Are data about previous admissions, ambulant treatment periods, and visits to emergency rooms readily available? Are data on previous diagnosis, about treatments, about dispositions, about family constellations readily at hand? No, they are not. They are retrievable in some cases, but only for those who really persevere. It often takes weeks before they arrive, and when they do arrive, they often are disappointing. Assuming that a record is legible, the records are frequently meager, fragmentary, and not systematized. That state of affairs detracts considerably from continuity of care and, consequently, from quality of care, the more so because many patients wander from one institution to another, from one clinic to another. If they stay with one clinic they often are treated by ever-changing generations of residents.

For such a department, a computerized tracking system and eventually a computerized record system would provide an important contribution to the resolution of the problem. Computers, however, though around now for a number of decades, have so far been profoundly underutilized in psychiatry, both in this country and in Europe. This is partly because of legitimate concerns about confidentiality of certain very personal data; partly because of illegitimate unwillingness to render a full account of one's diagnostic conclusions, therapeutic interventions, and their outcome; and partly, no doubt, because of shyness vis-à-vis a machinery that is still rather unfamiliar for many.

The department I invited you to imagine is actually not an imaginary one. It is our department of psychiatry here in the Albert Einstein College of Medicine/Montefiore Medical Center. We do realize the enormous potential of computers in contributing to quality of psychiatric care, in particular for that large contingent of chronically ill and chronically relapsing patients for which we are responsible. We felt the need to discuss our problems, our needs, our expectations, and our plans with a panel of experts. We wanted, moreover, to be informed about other possible applications of computers in psychiatry. Those were the reasons to organize this symposium. I am sincerely appreciative to David Baskin, who brought the idea into practice. Since we reasoned that our departmental problems were not unique, but symptomatic for the profession at large, we decided to organize, instead of a closed intradepartmental workshop, an open symposium, which we hope will help inform a wider range of mental health professionals concerned with these problems and with the welfare of their patients.

2

AN OVERVIEW OF ISSUES REGARDING CLINICAL APPLICATIONS IN PSYCHIATRY AND PSYCHOLOGY

David Baskin

About 20 or 30 years ago large mental health organizations and psychiatric hospitals with management information systems began using computers, at that time mainframe computers, large IBMs or other systems, in order to collect data, analyze what was happening to their patients, and determine characteristics of their patients.

With the advent of microcomputers, we have seen a tremendous change in the way small facilities and even private practitioners are approaching the whole issue of billing, analysis of data, and other related tasks. With the microcomputers, people are using word processing and Lotus 1–2–3 programs, and they are using the microcomputers to store and administer psychological tests as well. This has created quite a change in the way we are approaching the whole field of psychiatry and psychology. In academic environments, computers have been very much used in research for statistical analysis. Even SPSS, which is one of the most commonly used statistical packages, now comes in an abridged form so that one

5

could use it with a microcomputer. Computers have been used also for the simulation of patient and therapist responses, for didactic functions, as an adjunct in a research framework, even experimentally to see whether one can diagnose with a computer and how accurate it is relative to clinical judgments.

With the microcomputers we are finding tremendous flexibility in the way we can program our own systems. We are not dependent upon programmers or systems analysts, but can write our own programs and do any analyses in any of the functions we have mentioned. This flexibility plus the control of the data and the confidentiality (which does not exist when you send out data to be analyzed by a service bureau or you are connected via a dumb terminal to some large mainframe that may be miles away from your locale) are sustained through the use of microcomputers. The issue of confidentiality of patient data is solved when you have a microcomputer and you are the only person with access to these data.

What are the changes that will occur as a function or consequence of this computer revolution? What are the psychological effects of this computer revolution? Will therapists be replaced by the ideal computer? We now have banking by computer; are we going to have something like therapy by computer? We can now program responses of the computer on an experimental basis; people may be familiar with Eliza, which simulates the therapist's response to a patient's comments. Perhaps in the future, if you want a Gestalt therapist, you may be able to call a particular number and get a Gestalt computer. Are we going to see an increased withdrawal of people as a function of this computer revolution, concomitant with the revolution of technology that allows people to have many of their needs satisfied in their own homes?

Dr. Salamon, Director of Sound View-Throgs Neck Community Mental Health Center, has been investigating the whole issue of whether with computers people will be more open in disclosing data about themselves that may be relevant to their clinical treatment. He hypothesized that people may feel more open and free in disclosing information when they are not face to face with an individual. Of course, one may hypothesize the converse—that people when confronted with a computer may be aroused by paranoia and may be reluctant to respond openly.

We are very excited at Einstein about the possibility of developing a patient-tracking system. Not only will this system improve clinical care, it will also provide better follow-up of patients, and it will alert caretakers to information about patients, instead of their waiting for weeks until discharge data are transmitted. If you were the new therapist, you would immediately know critical data about the patient. It would also alert you as the caretaker on both sides of the system (discharging and admitting agency) when a patient is not showing up, so that we could then follow up and see what has happened. We could to some extent respond at an elementary level to the whole question of the proverbial revolving door. We are also excited about this from a research point of view, because we feel that a patient tracking system would be a great resource for epidemiological data. The Einstein College of Medicine family now renders 75% of psychiatric service visits and care to the mental health patients in the Bronx.

Professionals with an expertise in psychology, psychiatry, and computers are often asked, what computer should I buy? The first question is what functions they are going to be using the computer for. Very often I find that people are purchasing systems only because they feel that this is the bandwagon and they should hop aboard. Yet you can sometimes save $3,000 by purchasing a pack of index cards for 69¢, which will perform the same function that you have in mind. So, in addition to discussing aspects of computerization, the contributors will also be addressing the issue of limitations of their particular systems and limitations of computers in general. They will not be giving a global go-ahead of computerization without a determination of the real needs.

PART II

CLINICAL APPLICATIONS OF COMPUTERS

3

CLINICAL APPLICATIONS OF COMPUTERS: AN OVERVIEW

Marc D. Schwartz

In order to provide an idea of how computers are being used in clinical settings, the findings of a survey that was carried out with subscribers to *Computers in Psychiatry/Psychology* in 1986 will be presented in this chapter.

Computer technology has changed over the past few years. Not too long ago, the computer was a solution in search of a problem. Many people knew how computers were being used in large organizations and recognized their potential, but they did not have a clear idea of how to use a computer in mental health. Mental health professionals are now beginning to develop a better idea of what they want to do. The impediment at present seems to be finding the proper software and support to make sure the system functions efficiently.

In our survey we found, first of all, that the most frequently used software was not specifically mental health software, but generic word processing, database, and, to a certain extent, spread sheet software. Word processors have been used mainly for writing reports, articles, and papers. A relatively small number of clinicians have been using the word processor to record progress notes. The number is small because it takes an unusually dedicated clinician to sit down after each session and get the word processor going. It is also questionable how valuable such a process is. In using the computer, one would hope to have a very significant return on one's time investment. For example, a device like the CAT scanner requires a relatively small amount of time of the professional to get a very large amount of useful information from the system. The best applications of computers are those in which one's time and effort are minimal, while the amount of information one gets is very large.

The word processor was also used by some clinicians as an idea organizer. There has been a new genre of word processing software developed in the past two years, pioneered by a program called Think Tank, which allows one to write an outline and then zoom in on particular points and headings in the outline and expand upon them. One can zoom back at any time and see the full list of subheadings or the main headings.

The second most commonly used type of software in the survey was database programs. Database programs are used primarily to store, sort, search, and retrieve information. Mental health clinicians are using database programs to store and retrieve general information about patients. They are also using them for storing literature references and information about their reading, so that they can quickly retrieve citations they are looking for. One of the advantages that a database program offers is that it can do statistical analyses of data very, very quickly. People are also using database programs for billing, for preparing insurance forms, and for carrying out a variety of other functions.

Psychological testing programs were used by about one-third of the respondents to the survey. Almost half of the testing programs used were produced by Human Edge Software, a commercial company that does not sell specifically to mental health clinicians, but rather sells to the general public. Yet many mental health clinicians are using their products. Why? They are smoothly written programs that are easy to use, are readily available by mail or in a computer store, and do not cost a lot of money.

The other kinds of psychological testing programs used by survey respondents were MMPI programs, the WISC, and the WAIS. These products were available from a number of mental health software vendors.

Other applications mentioned by one or two subscribers were artificial intelligence, simulations, and biofeedback.

What kind of psychiatrist is using computers? It seems that mental health microcomputer users are dedicated and interested in technology; they are willing to experiment, ready to spend many evenings learning a new skill, and willing to put up with all kinds of problems when the system does not work right. They are often willing to develop their own programs. We are still in the era of the pioneer in many ways in the mental health computer field. The people who are developing programs often are innovative, eager to explore and to accept challenges.

The programs that are most useful are those that can be modified to a specific user's application. Those programs that are unmodifiable are not quite as useful to clinicians. Clinicians' practices vary so much from individual to individual, from geographical site to site, that there will always need to be some tailoring of programs in our field.

The question has come up as to why computers have not been more rapidly accepted in mental health settings. There is a debate whether this represents some conservatism on the part of mental health clinicians or whether there is something about the field that is not conducive to the use of technology. I run an educational technology company, and we were asked to do a study at a major corporation to determine why, after they purchased 12,000 IBM PCs, the computers were not being used in a productive way. This was an insurance company, and insurance companies, as you know, make heavy use of mainframe computers.

We did a study of the company, interviewing about 200 employees to try to determine what was behind the fact that these beautiful, shiny personal computers were gathering dust. One of the reasons my company was hired to do this study was that the insurance company believed that their employees might have a kind of psychological block against computer use. We found no psychological block. In fact, most people were quite eager to use the computer. What they needed to know, however, was what programs were available to do which tasks in each individual's particular line of work. Over and over again we heard, "If you will just give me the program and tell me how to use it." It is true that in the field of psychiatry many believe that the computer could be useful. What is not so clear are the answers to the following questions: What programs will be most helpful in our work? Which will make us more productive and/or more helpful to our patients? Where can we get them? and How do we get them to work?

How to get them to work is a major issue. Computers and programs tend to break down and have bugs in them. They require support for the hardware and education for their use. They require access to a kind of guru, someone who knows about a particular program and its idiosyncrasies. They require training. They require group support, in which people can share common problems. In the absence of an infrastructure supporting the users, microcomputers will not be used effectively and will not be adopted in a widespread manner. The issue of training and support has not been adequately dealt with. A great deal more needs to be done.

What kinds of mental health computer programs are available? The computer is being used extensively in a number of institutions for diagnosis and assessment. However, no matter how much work one does on computer diagnosis, there is a limitation to its value set by the reliability and validity of the diagnostic system. A computer program cannot be any better than the system it is based upon.

However, the computer can be very effective in gathering information from clinicians and/or patients, which can be very time saving, especially if one has a large number of patients.

I do not believe the computer will ever receive widespread use in small practices. But if a clinician has hundreds or thousands of patients being seen in the course of a year, an automated system will enhance his or her ability to gather information from those patients, not only for assessment, but also for maintenance and follow-up.

In a project that I have been involved in recently, a telephone connected to a computer does automated follow-up with patients. We are currently in a research stage, but I anticipate that we will develop a system that will actually be used in a clinical setting. The computer uses a digitized voice. It is able to either telephone an individual or to be called. The system asks by voice certain questions, such as whether the patient is taking his or her medication or following certain treatment prescriptions. The patient answers the questions by pressing buttons on the touchtone telephone. The computer is able to analyze those tones and branch to ask the next set of questions, depending upon the previous answers given. When there are large numbers of patients to be followed, it is generally difficult to find adequate staff to make those many telephone calls necessary to do the follow-up. We have been looking at automated phone systems for health promotion and illness prevention programs, as well as for following up on patients' use of medication.

With regard to psychiatrists' use of computers for psychological testing, in psychiatry we find ourselves in a somewhat awkward position. There is a plethora of computerized psychological tests available, yet most psychiatrists have never received adequate training in the use of them. Nevertheless, many psychiatrists are beginning to use these computerized tests without adequate training or without understanding their construction or interpretation. It is very important that test results be viewed not as the given truth. A clinician familiar with both the tests and the patient should always have an opportunity to see the test results before the clinician uses them to make diagnoses or recommendations.

Many current tests are old wine in new bottles—the old testing technology spruced up and put into a computer with a fancy printout. I look forward to the development of new kinds of testing programs that will truly capitalize on the computers' special capabilities. Computers can, for example, track the steps of an individual's problem-solving strategies. With a hypothetical problem that is to be solved in a three-minute period, a conventional test might indicate only the solution reached by the person being tested. One would not know what went on during the problem-solving process, what kind of problem-solving path the individual had taken, or what kind of deficits were present. Many individuals might reach the same end point but might have followed entirely different paths. Thus one of the interesting things about new types of computer tests is that they are able to track an individual's attempts at problem solving over time. Time itself is a variable that is easily measured by a computer. If an individual is given a multistep task to solve, the computer is able to determine how long it took to solve each step along the way.

Today relatively few clinicians are using the computer as a psychotherapy adjunct. The computer tends to be most useful in psychotherapy when used in the treatment of fairly focal disorders, such as desensitization treatment of a particular phobia. In these circumstances, where it is possible to program the computer to take the patient in a structured course through treatment, the computer gives results that are comparable to those obtained by a trained psychotherapist.

Another way in which the computer is being used is by providing enhanced video games for assisting with cognitive rehabilitation of patients who have had a cerebral accident or disorder. Most readers are familiar with the ubiquitous arcade game Pacman. Imagine someone who has had a stroke and who is just beginning to regain cognitive and physical abilities being faced with a vastly slowed-down version of Pacman and being able to move Pacman around the screen at a speed adjusted to the patient's ability. This approach can engage patients in an exercise effort that helps them regain some of their lost capabilities. It is an extremely tedious task for a rehabilitation therapist to provide training to these patients over a period of many months. There is good evidence to suggest that the use of these games is helpful, both with motoric coordination and with the ability to deal with concepts and words.

Another example of how the computer has been used in practice is with fantasy games. There is a class of computer programs that presents the player with a scenario on the screen: "You are living in the year 1200 and are trying to get from one castle to another. You face a long trek through a forest wilderness. . . ." The computer spells out the scenario in text on the screen. The player is accompanied by a group of fantasy companions—maybe a seer, a fighter, and a magical animal. He comes across certain challenges and problems: the bridge is blown away; a monster attacks the group; a strange cave needs to be explored. The screen states exactly what the player's choices are in dealing with these situations. These games have been used to assist adolescents with impulse control, with long-term planning, and with peer relationships. The therapist sits with the adolescent while the adolescent plays the game, and at a certain point will engage the adolescent in a dialogue about the game and about the decisions, in order to assist the player in making better decisions and developing restraints on impulsivity. Adolescents are excited about coming in to therapy to play these games, even though they may initially have resisted the whole notion of being in treatment. The main resistance to the use of these games comes from professionals who feel that it is somehow demeaning to play such games in the course of psychotherapy.

Another application of computers has been in the area of quality assurance. Here the computer monitors the kinds of therapeutic activities that take place in a unit or within a practice and points out areas in which the level of practice has not been up to certain standard levels of care. Reports and reminders are generally sent to clinicians. These systems seem to work very well in bringing up the level of care; but as soon as they are discontinued, the level of care slowly falls and, in not too many months, returns to the previous lower level. When the clinician is planning and budgeting mental health systems within his or her facility, it is important to bear in mind that long-term planning is absolutely essential and that the long-term, continuous investment of time and effort into the system is necessary for it to be successful.

The computer has often been used as a consultant and expert system. There are a number of computer programs currently available that can run on an Apple computer or an IBM PC that will tell the user about drug interactions. Once the names of the two drugs that one is thinking of prescribing for a patient are typed in, the program will search through its database and will state whether there is an interaction between the medications, what that interaction might be and what level of danger it poses for the patient.

Another computer project that I am carrying out provides a continuing medical education program for the American Psychiatric Association. APA members get a textbook about psychopharmacology, accompanied by a questionnaire and an answer sheet. In the past, members mailed the answer sheet to the association, where it was scored and then, a few weeks later, mailed back with a corrected answer sheet and suggestions for additional readings. That system was too slow. By the time members received their corrected questionnaire, they often had forgotten some of the questions.

Now members can call a toll-free number. A computer answers and asks for their APA membership number. It then gives instructions on how to proceed, requesting the answer to the first multiple-choice question. Members touchtone their answer and the system tells them whether their answer is correct and offers them the opportunity to hear an explanation of the correct answer or a literature reference. This system gives clinicians immediate feedback on their answers as well as useful references.

Self-help programs are another area where computers have been used. These programs have received quite a lot of attention and some notoriety, especially one for the treatment of sexual problems, and in particular one for men who were having difficulty with erections. The computer's video screen gave programmed instruction on how to deal with performance anxiety.

The Connecticut Psychiatric Society Committee on the Use of Computers drafted some general principles that computer users in psychiatry should bear in mind as they begin introducing computers and other technology into their practices. From the draft of this document:

1. A psychiatrist must maintain full professional responsibility for all consequences of the use of technology in his or her clinical or administrative practice. This responsibility must be borne both in direct clinical diagnosis and care and in the participation and use of the more broadly based information systems.

   We felt that this is an important principle to state because it is very easy to lose track of who is responsible for a clinically oriented computer system. A professional who has mental health training should have that responsibility. It should not be diffused into the hands of administrators and other people who do not have mental health training.

2. In introducing technology into practice, the psychiatrist should exercise the same level of care as in introducing any other type of clinical intervention or administrative procedure, such as a new drug, the use of peer review, and so forth. The psychiatrist should appropriately consider, alone or with the patient, the real and fantasy implications of these procedures, ascertain that they cause no harm, and use the usual precepts of scientific practice including the weighing of risks and benefits, permission to experiment, when warranted, publication of results, review by peers, etc.

3. The introduction of new technology is justified to increase the scope and quality of care by rendering it more effective, more economical, or better able to reach a wider range of patients. It is acceptable only if it maintains or raises the quality of care rendered, not if it dilutes or degrades it.

4. Psychiatrists should be knowledgeable about the opportunities and problems in the nature of electronically stored and accessed information.

5. Special care should be taken that the confidentiality of patient information is appropriately respected and guarded.

4

COMPUTERS AND PSYCHIATRIC DIAGNOSIS

John H. Greist

As recently as eight years ago, the panel on computing at the American Psychiatric Association annual meetings often outnumbered the audience. By now computers have become a part of the history of progress in medicine and not simply public nuisances or symbols of our age of alienation. Many of us idealized the turn of the century as a time when a renaissance physician such as William Osler could encompass most if not all of the facts of clinical medicine and use them to the patient's advantage. Osler succeeded in large part by *not* treating because he felt that physicians were as likely as not to harm patients with available remedies.

By the 1920s, complexity in medicine had increased and there was recognition of the need for documentation in hospital records of our evaluations, decisions and treatments. In our outpatient practices we could still use our memories. My father, who began practice in 1929, describes a distinguished older surgeon who was very put out by and very resistant to this innovative demand for record keeping. Finally, he was told he could not admit any additional patients until he kept written records. In obvious exasperation he scribbled fiercely on the chart of an appendectomy patient, and everyone went to see what the great man had written. They found, "Little by little and bit by bit, God in his mercy is healing this slit." This sort of passive-aggressive engagement with the requirements we face for documentation of the facts of medicine remains common.

We are all aware of the increasing complexity in medicine that led to specialization and subspecialization, and we frequently consult our colleagues in other specialties for help with problems outside our areas of expertise. As an example, in internal medicine there are over one million facts that an internist might need to use in evaluating and treating patients with the disorders within her purview. In psychiatry, we now have over 18,000 citations to the medical uses of lithium on file in our Lithium Information Center. There is no way we can even find relevant citations without using computers to help us.

The increasing complexity that we face across all of medicine requires computers to help us organize the facts for our use. Computers are particularly helpful in areas where they provide necessary structure for our efforts in specialization. Computers are much less helpful at the triage point, where clinical experience and even intuition are of greatest importance.

Some people in our generation will continue to practice without computers, and this is particularly true of traditional dynamic psychotherapists. Some physicians worry that computers may make only trivial suggestions, although a prescription for two aspirin may not be a trivial suggestion if it spares the patient a more noxious nostrum. Some anticipate that computers will complicate practice, and in fact that does happen. They can provide new information that you do not know what to do with. There is fear that computers will invade previously sacrosanct domains and usurp functions. Some rightfully object to the difficulties of using computers, which can at times be very challenging. Advertisers emphasize the user-friendliness of their programs, but there are programs that are user-hostile.

Microcomputers are accelerating the pace of change in the use of computers and the pace of acceptance simply because we are growing more familiar with computing. Even if adults have not bought them, their children have begun to use them in the schools. Those of us who began with batch processing on mainframes found that environment uncongenial. Time-shared minicomputers were fine, but only a few had access to them. Almost everyone can have access to microcomputers. More than 14 million microcomputers were sold in the United States in 1988. Prices continue to drop at the same time that performance increases, a unique commodity in medicine. Robert Noyce, inventor of the semiconductor, wrote in *Scientific American* over a decade ago that the microcomputer, then available at a cost of perhaps $300,

> has more computing capacity than ENIAC, the first large electronic computer. It is twenty times faster, has a larger memory, is thousands of times more reliable, consumes the power of a light bulb rather than a locomotive, occupies one thirty-thousandth the volume and costs one ten-thousandth as much. (Noyce, 1977, p. 65)

Christopher Evans wrote a charming little book in 1979 entitled *The Micro Millenium*, and gave other trenchant examples of the increase in computing performance. He stated:

> If the efficiency and cheapness of the car had improved at the same rate as the computer over the last two decades, a Rolls Royce would cost about $3.00, would get three million miles to the gallon, and would deliver enough power to drive the QE II. (p. 76)

> Thirty years ago a computer with the same number of functions as the human brain would have had to be the size of New York City and would have used more power than the subway system. Today that computer would be the size of a T.V. set. By the end of the eighties, it will be as small as the human brain and will run on a transistor radio battery. (p. 76)

In just ten years the machines have attained the intelligence level of an earwig, an unimpressive accomplishment, until one realizes that it took man's ancestors several million centuries to make the same leap. (p. 76)

In addition to the increased availability, affordability and performance of microcomputers, we have much better products now than before, beginning with languages and operating systems. While some are waiting to see if UNIX is going to mature on the microcomputer, MUMPS has arrived on the microcomputer (see Chapter 10 for more information about MUMPS). I recommend the several good MUMPS operating systems for your consideration.

Applications written in these languages are becoming more and more useful and easier to use. Developing them is slow work, and properly evaluating their validity and reliability is challenging. Keeping programs current is an unending task. This entire process is accelerating because more and more people are using computers. Each user can potentially develop a program that meets his or her personal needs and can then contribute that program to the profession's general armamentarium.

Documentation, if it existed at all, used to be a terrible problem. While sometimes still poor, documentation is steadily improving and some is even available on-line, so users don't have to go back and forth between their computer and a book to know how to use it. Perhaps the best widespread example of excellent on-line documentation is the Apple Macintosh with its mouse and the screen icons.

With regard to terminals, we have the familiar video display that is quite adequate for most of our needs. In spite of the fact that there are mice, light pens, and finger touching, none of those terminals has really surpassed the keyboard and video display for general purpose computing. When we reach the point that we can speak and the computer will understand what we have said and speak to us in reply, that will become an interface that will challenge the video display keyboard terminal for inexperienced users. Until then, our old standby, the video display terminal, is likely to remain the dominant means of interacting with the computer.

We need computers in clinical medicine because we face problems that we cannot solve with our present resources and techniques. Computers will help us close the gap between what is known and what is practiced, and they facilitate problem-solving learning. What we learn in the process of solving a clinical problem is often long remembered. What we read in textbooks as students is often forgotten after the examination.

We have an available technology, the cost of the technology is decreasing, the quality and quantity of applications is increasing, and we have a growing understanding of the role of the computer, not as a competitor, but as an aid to our abilities, providing help wherever we need structure and specialized information.

COMPUTERS IN PSYCHIATRIC DIAGNOSIS

Psychiatric diagnosis is one area in which computers are beginning to be clinically helpful. Diagnosis is clearly the cornerstone of enlightened practice. There are many reasons we need to diagnose and do it well. We diagnose to make prognoses, to select treatments, to communicate among ourselves, and to find homogeneous populations for research. We are trained to diagnose by taking histories, doing physical examinations, using selected laboratory tests, and following the course of an illness, and to obtain consultation when we are uncertain about diagnosis. If we are trained to be expert diagnosticians, why do we need help from a machine? There are a number of reasons.

Most readers will be familiar with the evolution of psychiatric diagnosis in the United States over the last 30 or more years. The first edition of *The Diagnostic and Statistical Manual of the American Psychiatric Association* was published in 1952. *DSM-I* reflected a rather Meyerian approach to diagnosis and lasted 16 years until 1968, when it was succeeded by *DSM-II*. *DSM-II* was 134 pages long, and had a substantial emphasis on unverifiable etiologic factors in diagnosis. The reliabilities that clinicians could obtain in describing patients were low, and attempts to use *DSM-II* in computer diagnostic systems, such as those developed by John Overall, Leo Hollister, Bob Spitzer, and Jean Endicott, failed not because the computer contribution was poor, but because the diagnostic system itself was so unreliable.

About this time workers at Washington University developed specific criteria for diagnosis, which appeared in 1972 in *The Archives of General Psychiatry*. Subsequently Jean Endicott and Bob Spitzer developed the Research Diagnostic Criteria, which evolved from the Washington University work and were published in 1978. After substantial debate, *DSM-III* emerged in 1980, 494 pages long. We are all familiar with its multiaxial approach and the nonetiologic descriptive emphasis of *DSM-III*. Although it is a large step forward, with reliabilities that are at least double what we had with *DSM-II*, *DSM-III* is so complicated that it is really beyond our capacity to use it properly. In *DSM-III-R* we see a progressive decrease from 16 to 12 to 7 years between new classifications, reflecting a greater interest in diagnosis that is going to have a payoff in all domains of clinical psychiatry. Consider the complexity of the flow diagrams for the Research Diagnostic Criteria, which are hard enough for humans to process. *DSM-III* and *DSM-III-R* are almost an order of magnitude larger. I readily admit my need for help with the complex structure of *DSM-III* and *DSM-III-R*.

Why do we need structure in diagnosis? Kiernan et al. (1976), evaluating first-year Maudsley psychiatric registrars when they are at their compulsive best, found many failures to collect important information and record it in the charts. Weitz found that physicians recorded the 15 mental status items that had been identified as being so important that they should be included in every initial examination in only 4 out of 49 cases they examined. When the same physicians used a checklist for the 15 items, with the same patients, they recorded all 15 items in all 49 patients. Structure certainly yielded completeness, but relevance may be more important; clinicians may be skillfully separating grain from chaff.

In another study, Climent reviewed the incidence of suicidal thoughts, delusions of control, and significant weight loss as recorded in the patient's chart. He found that they were respectively 3 times, 10 times, and 50 times more likely to be captured when clinicians used a structured checklist than with a free-form clinical interview.

In a study we conducted of a computer interview in an emergency room to elicit symptoms relevant to trauma, infections and psychiatric problems, we found that the doctors, nurses and clinical staff often failed to document the presence or absence of allergy to penicillin, even when patients were given parenteral penicillin. We also found that the clerk registering patients made errors in spelling 10 of the 30 patients' names, while only one error was made when the computer terminal was used by the patient. At Washington University, St. Louis, residents processed the Feighner criteria based on data collected using the Renard structured interview and failed to make indicated diagnoses 19% of the time (false negatives) and made unjustified diagnoses 18% of the time (false positives). This led Lee Robins and John Helzer (1981) to process all of the Diagnostic Interview Schedule logic by computer.

COMPUTER CONSULTATION IN PSYCHIATRY

Some of the best indicators of where we are heading come from medicine and surgery. Howard Bleich and Warner Slack run the Computer Medicine Laboratory at the Beth Israel Hospital in Boston, and I recommend their article describing the Beth Israel computer system, which appeared in the March 21, 1985, *New England Journal of Medicine*. The Beth Israel Hospital Information System is, in my view, the best large-scale computer medicine application that has been done anywhere in the world.

Howard Bleich (1974) also developed a fluid, electrolyte, and acid-base abnormality program in the late sixties. This program asks doctors to describe electrolytes, relevant patient history, physical findings, and laboratory results. It takes two or three minutes for the physician to provide this information to the program; the computer then solves the Henderson-Hasselbach equation, a quadratic equation difficult for the clinician to do in her head. The computer provides an evaluation note with a differential diagnosis and suggestions for treatment. In 1974, Howard reported on an evaluation of that program against 21 questions from a physician's self-assessment examination and compared the computer results with those obtained by physicians who restricted their practice to nephrology. The computer outperformed 98% of those subspecialists. It missed one question out of 21, dealing with the effect of an extract of licorice on potassium levels. The computer was promptly reprogrammed to deal with that issue correctly, has been updated since that time, and is one of the programs available on line for use by all doctors at the Beth Israel Hospital. When I was chief resident in medicine in 1969–1970, I used that program for consultation with difficult problems in that area, and it was better than I was then, and it is surely even further ahead now.

DeDombal (1979), working in England with consultant surgeons, developed a program that dealt with 11 causes of abdominal pain and found that the surgeons improved their diagnostic accuracy from 81% to 91% when the program was in use. The magnitude of improvement may not seem very great, but it meant that the number of perforated appendixes decreased from 36% to 4%. At the same time the number of false negative laporotomies decreased from 25% to 7%, and this happened while the number of discharges in the first 24 hours was increasing. Here again is a program that has clear clinical impact.

McDonald (1976), working in Indiana at a chronic disease medicine clinic where congestive heart failure, diabetes, rheumatoid arthritis, and hypertension are treated, asked doctors practicing in the clinic to specify the protocols by which they wanted to practice medicine. He then monitored their performance and found they were complying with 20% of their own protocols. He put a computer reminder system into effect that, for example, would remind the doctor of the rule about ordering a blood sugar in a diabetic patient who develops an infection. With reminders, physician compliance with their own protocols rose to 50%. Why didn't it go to 100%? McDonald (1976) talked about the nonperfectibility of man (I'm sure he didn't intend to exclude women). There are things that humankind has difficulty doing, and there are limits to what we can do on our own. When that reminder program was removed, the physicians' compliance with their own protocols fell to baseline.

For problems in internal medicine, Miller, Myers, and Pope (1982) have been working on Caduceus. The accuracy of Caduceus is not as high as that achieved by Bleich's (1974) and DeDombal's (1979) programs, probably because Caduceus deals with a broader domain of problems that are difficult to treat as fully.

If we consider *DSM-III* consultation, a problem more germane to mental health, we all recognize the screening question for psychosis and mood disorders. In this case, the clinician indicates that there is a depressed, irritable, or expansive mood by pressing the number-two key. When this key is pressed, the computer branches to the question about depressed mood or loss of interest or pleasure. The branching takes the clinician through the shortest path, so that all the relevant areas are covered without redundancy. Next, the computer displays the B criteria for major depression. A number of responses are made; they can be made in any order. It is easy to change answers and it is possible to back up to previous displays to change answers. This program, written by Harold Erdman in our computing laboratory, makes *DSM-III* diagnoses very accurately for all diagnoses, including those of children and for all disorder subtypes. We have tested this program with medical students, and they like it very much because it helps them learn *DSM-III*. We have tried to have residents use it, and some do during their first year, when they will do most anything we tell them to do. Then their participation flags. It takes only 10 minutes for the doctor to interact with the computer. We do not understand this low use completely, but we are sure that at some level it is because there still is not enough of a penalty for making the wrong diagnosis or not enough payoff for making better diagnoses. Behavior is shaped by its consequences.

All evidence indicates that structure contributes to diagnostic accuracy. We felt that patients might be able to provide the symptom data needed for diagnosis.

COMPUTER USE IN INTERVIEWING

When the Feighner criteria were published, workers at Washington University in St. Louis realized that it was difficult for clinicians to collect necessary diagnostic data in an unstructured clinical interview. The Renard Interview Schedule (Helzer et al., 1981) was developed to help clinicians structure their questioning for diagnostic information necessary to make Feighner criteria diagnoses. The

Schedule for Affective Disorders and Schizophrenia (SADS) served a similar purpose for the Research Diagnostic Criteria. The Diagnostic Interview Schedule (DIS) was developed to make a subset of *DSM-III* diagnoses from data collected by lay interviewers. This interview was used in the epidemiologic catchment area studies that were reported in the October 1984 *Archives of General Psychiatry*. Bob Spitzer, Janet Williams, and colleagues (1988) also developed the Structured Clinical Interview for *DSM-III-R* (SCID). In contrast to the DIS, the SCID requires clinical judgment.

We were interested in the DIS because if lay interviewers could administer it without clinical judgment, there was the possibility that a computer could administer it as well. With very slight modifications, we programmed our minicomputer to directly interview psychiatric patients. We have recently prepared the program to run under the MUMPS Standard Operating System available on IBM XT and AT and compatible microcomputers.

The history of computer interviewing began at the University of Wisconsin when Warner Slack (1966) first used a classic LINC computer built by Joseph Hind, a professor in the neurophysiology department. Questions appeared on a tiny cathode ray tube in a flickering four-by-six dot matrix, and patients pressed keys on a modified typewriter keyboard. Questions and responses were stored on tapes, and patients were interviewed in front of the computer console with all its lights blinking. Summaries of the interviews were printed on a 10-character-per-second teletype. The computer taught patients how to control the interview with a very interactive teaching section and it invoked humor (some of it quite juvenile) as a means of establishing rapport.

In our work the DIS was faithfully presented, using the same probes that human interviewers would follow to determine the significance of a symptom acknowledged by the patient. Thus, for a response indicating weight loss, the computer would follow up by asking whether a doctor had been told about the weight loss. If the answer was yes, it would then determine what the doctor had stated regarding the probable cause of the weight loss.

Completion times for inpatients averaged two hours and for outpatients one hour and 15 minutes, which is related both to the greater number of symptoms described by inpatients and the severity of their psychopathology.

Immediately after the interview was completed, the computer printed a summary for the clinician. This included diagnoses and the detailed patient responses to *DSM-III* criteria on which diagnoses were based. The clinician could quickly scan the summary and compare the data obtained by the computer with his or her own impressions. There was also a patient summary that we provided to our patients. The patient summary did not provide diagnoses, but indicated the items the patients acknowledged. This was helpful to us in validating the responses they made and was also quite popular with patients.

The design of our study involved random assignment of 150 psychiatric patients to receive either the computer or a human DIS first. This was then followed by the alternative form of presentation, so that each patient received two DIS interviews, one presented by a human and one by the computer. After a great number of analyses, I can summarize our findings by saying there is no difference between DISs collected by a computer and those collected by a trained human interviewer. When we compared diagnostic agreement between a DIS conducted *either* by a human or a computer with the clinical diagnoses obtained, the agreement was lower. In some instances, we feel it is clear that the clinician is more accurate, especially for affective and anxiety disorders; at other times, the computer appears more accurate, for example, in areas of alcohol and other drug abuse. Our conclusion is that if one wishes to conduct DIS interviews, there are advantages to computer administration. The costs are less, the computer is available at any time, is seldom "sick" and results in little, if any, interviewer burnout. When changes were made in the DIS, we upgraded the computer program. The continuing medical education of computers is easier than the continuing medical education of clinicians and lay interviewers.

How can the DIS, an instrument developed for epidemiologic research, be of use to a clinician? All patients coming to the Anxiety Disorders Center or the Center for Affective Disorders at the University of Wisconsin complete the DIS before they are seen.

About two-thirds of the time, the diagnoses clinicians made are included in the DIS summary, and that is gratifying. More exciting are disagreements with clinician diagnoses, which suggest either a need for improvements in the DIS or, perhaps one-quarter of the time, diagnoses that clinicians had overlooked. Patients are obtaining benefit from the DIS that they would not have obtained from the clinician alone.

To indicate the potential of structured interviewing and structured assistance with *DSM-III* diagnostic processing, we had two interviewers complete DISs on the same patient and then process them with Harold Erdman's *DSM-III* program (Greist et al., 1984). Kappa agreement with 49 complicated inpatients was .86; with two separate interviewers and more than 25 different inpatients a Kappa agreement of .80 was obtained.

Ken Mathisen at the Carrier Foundation has also been using the computer version of the DIS interview. He studied 135 psychiatric inpatients and compared their diagnoses with diagnoses of clinicians who were taking care of the patients. The Kappa agreements for Axis I disorders of .6 to .7 were as good as those found in the *DSM-III* field trials. Interestingly, we had a separate diagnostician who also examined the same patients (both of the clinicians had an average of 10 years of postresidency experience). The Kappa agreements between the two physicians were no better than those between the index physician and the computer.

There are limitations with DIS diagnoses, as there are with any diagnostic system. As we work with patients over a period of months or years, we continue to learn new things about them that improve the accuracy of our diagnostic formulations. It is unlikely that any single diagnostic interview will elicit all information relevant to diagnosing that patient. The computer interview does provide a compulsive psychiatric diagnostic system review in a way that humans cannot. It is inhumane to ask humans to become machines.

IMPLICATIONS OF COMPUTER INTERVIEWING

What about the effects of computer interviewing on rapport? Will computer interviews dehumanize psychiatry? Our experience suggests they will have the opposite effect. Computer interviews and paper-and-pencil questionnaires increase the amount of time that I have with the patient to try to understand their experience of being in the world rather than just to collect the symptoms they suffer from. Computer interviews provide us with better data and, at the same time, more time to understand the patient.

There is little systematic information on the issue of rapport, but Saghir (1971) found that the number of empathic statements made during structured interviews was equal to those made in free clinical interviews. The computer interview asks patients if they want to take a break, is programmed to be friendly and positively reinforcing, and tries hard not to boss patients or convey negative judgments. Strong opinions abound regarding the effects on rapport of note taking and consultation of texts in the presence of patients. Very little data exist to support or refute these opinions.

What about nonverbal data? There is no question that human interviewers can pick up nonverbal cues (such as inflections of speech, innuendos and gestures) that are important in the diagnostic process and that computers have great difficulty in perceiving, let alone interpreting. It is possible to have a computer interview branch contingent on response latency, so that if a patient responded unusually slowly to a particular question, the computer might branch to ask other questions about that issue. We have chosen not to pursue this type of branching logic, feeling that we have only begun to tap the potential of verbal information. Until we have made more progress in understanding verbal exchanges, the payoff from pursuit of nonverbal communication is unlikely to be worth the effort. We are not advocating either verbal data or nonverbal data and feel that every patient who has a computer interview should also be seen by a clinician who can pick up nonverbal cues.

What about confidentiality? This issue is decreasing in importance in clinicians' minds and has never been much of a problem for patients. More than a decade ago, we interviewed adolescents about illicit drug use and provided them with an option to "skip" a response. Less than 1% skipped questions about cocaine, marijuana, or alcohol abuse. In many of our interviews, we provide patients with an option to delete the entire interview after they complete it. At that point, they understand exactly what questions will be asked and what their answers have been. It is very difficult for a patient to erase information from a clinician's mind. We have also implemented an elaborate series of codes, passwords, and identifications that make it very difficult to gain entry to a computer system. At the Beth Israel Hospital in Boston, each user has a unique code and those codes are assigned to specific terminals. If a person has guessed or stolen an entry code and tries to use it at a terminal that is not programmed to accept it, the terminal beeps SOS 18 times and cannot be used until it is reset by a member of the computer staff. Data can also be encrypted and, while any code can be broken, the cost of doing so quickly becomes prohibitive. For our database management system written in MUMPS, we asked a very skilled MUMPS programmer to try to break in. After four days, he discerned how the encrypting system worked, but estimated it would take another week to break the code.

What about patient acceptance of computer interviewing? From the very beginning of computer interviewing to the present, patients have almost always enjoyed the experience, and some have preferred giving the kinds of information collected to a computer rather than to a human. Even those who dislike the experience usually give valid information. Psychiatric patients are not different from other medical patients. We also looked at the effect of repeated interviews over time on patient acceptance and found that it increased over the course of four identical interviews on dimensions of liking the interview, comfort, getting their ideas and feelings across, and the extent to which they felt the right questions were being asked and they could understand the questions. There are human factors that interfere with computer interviews and intellectual ability, advancing age, and visual acuity are three of them. In general, people under the age of 65 who have graduated from high school have little if any trouble with computer interviewing. On the positive side, computer interviews can be presented in whatever language the person prefers, with summaries being generated in the language of the clinician.

PSYCHIATRIC IMPLICATIONS OF COMPUTER INTERVIEWING

There are a number of other psychiatric applications of computer interviewing. Tony Carr and his colleagues (1981) working at the Institute of Psychiatry in London wrote questions for computer administration based on the Hamilton Depression Rating Scale. They were able to segregate depressed patients from normal controls, using a cutoff score of 10. While there were a few false-negative diagnoses using this cutoff, no false positives appeared.

We compared computer prediction of suicide risk based on information collected directly by computer from 63 psychiatric inpatients with thoughts of suicide with predictions made by clinicians caring for them. Patients were followed prospectively for 18 months. The computer significantly (P≤.001) outperformed the clinicians in predicting suicide attempts in the 12 individuals who made them. The computer's prediction was 84% chance of attempt, while the clinicians predicted a 31% chance. As is well known, the false-positive suicide attempt prediction rate is a limiting factor on the accuracy of suicide risk predictions. Still, when the problem domain under consideration is narrow, as in the case of suicide risk prediction, the computer outperforms clinicians.

Another computer interview developed at the University of Wisconsin collected target problem descriptions directly from patients. Using the full typewriter keyboard, patients describe their target problem in their own words. They also define the effects of the problem on their life and activities, what the problem is like at its worst, how they would be or act differently if the problem were solved, and the frequency and severity of the problem. Patients also rated themselves on the Hopkins Symptom Checklist, which provided a standardized measure of symptoms to complement the target problem approach. This interview was used on repeated occasions and was found to be highly acceptable to patients and to provide accurate and reliable measures of patient change. At this point in our clinic's history, we still do not have enough computing resources to use this program on line with all patients, but we do use a paper-and-pencil version of the SCL-90, which is scored by the computer and provides comparative summaries for all occasions the instrument was given.

COMPUTERS AS PSYCHOTHERAPISTS

While prophecy is often a substitute for accomplishment in clinical computing and many other domains—and we have heard expressions of both alarm and amazement regarding computer psychotherapy programs—I want to present data on two computer programs that do conduct effective psychotherapy. First is a program developed by Carr and Ghosh (1983b) at the Institute of Psychiatry.

They programmed a microcomputer to interview patients about phobic avoidance and to design a treatment prescription based on information the patient had provided. The computer prints the treatment prescription for the next week in terms of exposure sessions to be conducted, ratings of anxiety, coping tactics and comments. More than 70 patients were randomly assigned to be treated by the computer program, by Dr. Ghosh, who wrote the computer program, or by a self-help chapter from Isaac Marks's (1978) book, Living with Fear. There was no significant difference in treatment outcomes, either in ratings made by patients themselves or by researchers blind to treatment condition. We may take small comfort in knowing that there is a slight trend favoring the physician.

In our computing laboratory in Wisconsin, Paulette Selmi wrote her doctoral dissertation on a cognitive behavior therapy program for individuals with mild-to-moderate depression. Although these were volunteer recruits, many of them had previously failed to respond to other treatments (including antidepressant medication) for depression. Entry criteria were a chief complaint of depression or some synonym of depression; Beck depression scores above 16; SCL-90 depression cluster scores at or above the 65th percentile; Research Diagnostic Criteria diagnoses of major or minor depression; and depression of such severity that it was interfering with functioning in their self-defined major life role. These patients were symptomatically identical with our general psychiatric clinic outpatients. Computer-treated patients did as well as those treated by a well-trained human therapist; both treated groups did significantly better than the treatment-on-demand control group ($P \leq 0.001$). At two-month follow-up, the control group had regressed toward baseline, while both treated groups continued to improve. There was no significant difference in outcomes between the two treated groups. The transient improvement in the treatment-on-demand control group may have been related to the five-minute telephone contact Dr. Selmi made with those subjects each week to assess suicide risk.

I am indebted to David Servan-Schreiber for suggesting an analogy that may help us understand some of our feelings about the use of computers for psychotherapy. We can imagine music lovers at the turn of the century engaged in discussion of ways to disseminate great music to the masses. There would be controversy about the quality of music that might be produced in the provinces by nonprofessional orchestras as well as some criticism of the elitist nature of big-city orchestras which offered their superior performances at a cost that only a few could afford.

Debate about these issues was somewhat muted by the appearance of records, radio, television, and tape recordings of increasingly high fidelity. Still, detractors grumbled that these new technologies were not the "real thing," and they grew nostalgic about the importance of human contact between artists and their public, the atmosphere of the concert hall, and the pleasure each member of the audience derived from attending and paying a fee for listening to the great performance. These devotees were unlikely to acknowledge such advantages of home performances as lower cost, greater choice, constant availability, control of volume, and so on.

Some connoisseurs also expressed worry that the great orchestras and the prices they could charge grew in proportion to the dissemination of their performances.

At least computer therapies can be programmed not to seduce and sleep with their patients. The use of inhuman devices is not inhumane, although it will be ironic if the most human of all therapies is ultimately provided by computers.

ADDITIONAL COMPUTER USES

Finally, I would like to focus on our heavy use of the computer in the Lithium Information Center. We have over 18,000 citations to the medical uses of lithium, which are contained in a Lithium Library version of the Paper Chase Program. Citations can be found by any combination of author name, word in the title, journal, date span, or key word. Even when useful citations are found, most clinicians and lay persons do not have access to the articles or time to read them. We have written more than 100 synopses of clinically relevant subjects that we have culled from our reading of the literature. One person works full-time to keep this Lithium Index updated. A third interactive computer program is the Lithium Consultation, which permits clinicians to describe a patient and receive help with diagnosis, lithium treatment, and management of side effects.

We also make heavy use of the computer through a database management system, which is very important for our financial survival and other administrative purposes, including planning and patient accountability. Word processing has revolutionized the business of writing and, for academics, self-plagiarism is facilitated. We have noted as well that secretarial burnout and consequent turnover have been reduced.

Telecommunications are beginning to be useful as we connect with the Paper Chase front end for the National Library of Medicine's El Hill Database, which most of us have previously accessed through the Medline front end, which requires a medical librarian. We will also be using telecommunications for electronic mail and direct filing of insurance claims with insurance companies as a means of reducing turnaround time and accounts receivable. The present task is to integrate all of these functions into a usable system on microcomputers such as the IBM XT or AT or compatibles.

OVERCOMING RESISTANCE TO COMPUTER TECHNOLOGY

When computers first appeared, prophets thought they would quickly facilitate most aspects of the practice of medicine and psychiatry. In addition to many inherent limitations of the programs prepared by those working with computers, there has been resistance to the introduction of computers in medicine, particularly in psychiatry. What are the origins of inappropriate resistance to automation and innovation?

Computing is only the latest technology to encounter opposition. Examples from the transportation industry are legendary. The buggy whip manufacturers failed to realize that they were really in the business of catalyzing movement and, similarly, railroads held that they were simply in the business of railroading and overlooked the larger issue of the business of transportation. Resistance to new and efficient means of communication is not limited to physicians. Despite the great efficiencies offered by word processors and dictaphones, the *Wall Street Journal* reported in March, 1985, that only 1% of executive officers of large corporations use word processors and only 10% use dictaphones, while 89% use paper and pencil to write drafts of their letters.

At the end of his career, Max Planck (1949) commented, "A new scientific truth does not triumph by convincing its opponents and making them see the light, but rather because its opponents eventually die, and a new generation grows up that is familiar with it" (pp. 33–34). Charles Darwin (1859), at the conclusion of *On the Origin of Species*, wrote:

Although I am fully convinced of the truth of the views given in this volume . . . I by no means expect to convince experienced naturalists whose minds are stocked with a multitude of facts all viewed, during a long course of years, from a point of view directly opposite to mine. . . . But I look with confidence to the future—to young and rising naturalists, who will be able to view both sides of the question with impartiality. (pp. 295–296)

Thomas Kuhn (1962) has identified the basic human problem of accommodating shifts in paradigms. We continue to practice what we were preached because, in part, of the ordeal of change. As psychiatrists, we attempt to help our patients with their difficulties in making changes and it should not, but frequently does, surprise us when our colleagues have difficulty with change.

This sort of nihilism aside, what can we say about the process of adapting to innovation? In part, it depends on the goals of innovation and who is being affected by the innovations. If we are considering clinical computing innovations, such as treatment planning, drug exceptions reporting, diagnostic screening, or progress reports, those changes affect clinicians very directly. If we are planning administrative changes, such as agency planning, accountability, and financial programs, then another group is primarily affected. If we are anticipating computer programs for psychological testing, which can become routine, boring, and can lead to psychologist burnout, still another group is affected. If we are anticipating computer psychotherapy, different issues will arise. Resistance to innovation will clearly vary, depending on the group being asked to make changes and to use the programs. Clinicians often have substantial resistance to administrative programs which require increased paperwork on their part. Unless they get something back for their effort, why should they change their behavior? Clinicians are likely to view requests to provide additional data as an interference with both their clinical style and the time they have available for patient contact. On the other hand, clinicians would welcome aid with repetitive tasks such as psychological testing. Some clinicians will object strongly to the use of computers for therapy for a variety of reasons. Administrators are unlikely to object to changes, except to those that would reveal their limitations and affect their status or power.

If one considers the structural level of change, are individuals being asked to change their cognitive style? Do they have an intrinsic interest in programmatic functioning? Are they fascinated with computers and planning to make a career providing consultations about mental health computing or writing scholarly papers about computing? What is their personal philosophy about using computers? The text of some journals is now available on computers, but I still enjoy the visual and tactile process of receiving and reading the *New England Journal of Medicine* in paper form.

Within a group being asked to adapt to computers, goal conflicts are likely to emerge. Is someone going to be evaluated by someone new? What effect will the computer system have on the distribution of power and authority? It is interesting that when the Eastern Airlines employees were offered a position on the board of directors, they were pleased and accepted the position—but what they went to the mat for was the data contained in the Eastern Airlines computers. They recognized that data and the capacity to manipulate data are power. Our administrators may not want everyone to have access to the data on computers.

What about methods of communication? Are we going to be happy with electronic mail? It is true that we play telephone tag with each other, often over periods of days or even weeks. I know of one company using electronic mail that has an average communication time of two hours, including nights and weekends. On the other hand, many people enjoy meeting with colleagues in the coffee room to exchange information; the amount of important business that is transacted over coffee or lunch is impressive. It simply is not clear how new computer technologies will be used in mental health. Some will clearly be helpful and find their place, while others that offer great potential for improvement will fail because they are unacceptable to various mental health constituencies.

When I started in this area in 1967, I thought that almost every store would eventually sell computers. That has happened. I also thought that every doctor would have a computer in his or her office, but computers are now just beginning to appear in doctors' offices. Some doctors clearly fear being replaced, or worse, becoming mere appendages to computers or perhaps simply power sources for them. Still, I doubt that a variation of Skinner's aphorism will prevail: If a doctor can be replaced by a computer, he or she should be. Instead, I hope that we will find that behind every great man or woman stands a great computer. We are developing a growing capacity to use computer programs to complement our skills, abilities, and functions in areas where our inherent limitations interfere with the practice of the highest quality medicine.

REFERENCES

Bleich, H. L., R. F. Beckley, G. L. Horowitz, et al. 1985. Clinical computing in a teaching hospital. *New England Journal of Medicine* 312:756–764.

Bleich, H. L. 1974. Automated instructional programs for advanced medical education. In *Computers in biomedical research,* ed. R. W. Stacy and B. D. Waxman, vol. 4. New York and London: Academic Press.

Carr, A. C., A. Ghosh. 1983a. Accuracy of behavioural assessment by computer. *British Journal of Psychiatry* 142:66–70.

Carr, A. C. 1983b. Response of phobic patients to direct computer assessment. *British Journal of Psychiatry* 142:60–65.

Carr, A. C., A. Ghosh, R. J. Ancill, A. Margo. 1981. Direct assessment of depression by microcomputer. *Acta Psychiatrica Scandinavica* 64:415–422.

Climent, C. E., R. Plutchik, and H. Estrada. 1975. A comparison of traditional and symptom-checklist-based histories. *American Journal of Psychiatry* 132:450–453.

Darwin, C. 1859. *On the origin of species*. London: J. Murray.

DeDombal, F. T. 1979. Computers and the surgeon—a matter of decision. In *Surgery Annual*, ed. L. M. Nyhus, p. 33–57. New York: Appleton-Century Crofts.

Evans, C. 1980. *The micro millenium*. New York: The Telecom Library.

Feighner, J. P., E. Robins, S. B. Guze, R. A. Woodruff, G. Winokur, and R. Munoz. 1972. Diagnostic Criteria for use in psychiatric research. *Archives of General Psychiatry* 26:57.

Greist, J. H., K. S. Mathisen, M. H. Klein, L. S. Benjamin, et al. 1984. Psychiatric diagnosis: What role for the computer? *Hospital and Community Psychiatry* 35:1089–1093.

Greist, J. H., M. H. Klein, L. J. Van Cura, and J. Faulkner. 1977. Computer applications in psychiatry at the University of Wisconsin: Current status. *Current Concepts Psychiatry* 3:13–16.

Helzer, J. E., L. N. Robins, J. L. Krughan, et al. 1981. Renard diagnostic interview with R.D.I.: Its reliability and procedural validity with physicians and lay interviewers. *Archives of General Psychiatry* 38:393–398.

Kiernan, W. E. S., R. G. McCreadie, W. L. Flanagan. 1976. Trainees' competence in psychiatric case writing. *British Journal of Psychiatry* 129:167–172.

Kuhn, T. S. 1962. *The structure of scientific revolutions*. Chicago: The University of Chicago Press.

Marks, I. M. 1978. *Living with fear*. New York: McGraw Hill.

McDonald, C. J. 1976. Protocol-based computer reminders, the quality of care and the non-perfectibility of man. *New England Journal of Medicine* 295:194–198.

Miller, R. A., H. E. Pope, and J. D. Myers. 1982. Internist-1, an experimental computer-based diagnostic consultant for general internal medicine. *New England Journal of Medicine* 307:468–476.

Noyce, R. N. 1977. Microelectronics. *Scientific American* September: 62–70.

Planck, M. 1949. *Scientific autobiography and other papers*. New York: Philosophical Library.

Saghir, M. T. 1971. A comparison of some aspects of structured and unstructured psychiatric interviews. *American Journal of Psychiatry* 128:180–184.

Slack, W. V., and C. W. Slack. 1977. Talking to a computer about emotional problems; a comparative study. *Psychotherapy: Theory, Research and Practice* 14:156–164.

Slack, W. V. 1971. Computer-based interviewing system dealing with nonverbal behavior as well as keyboard responses. *Science* 171:84–87.

Slack, W. V., L. J. Van Cura, and J. H. Greist. 1970. Computers and doctors: Use and consequences. *Computers and Biomedical Research* 3:521–527.

Slack, W. V., and L. J. Van Cura. 1968. Patient reaction to computer-based medical interviewing. *Computers and Biomedical Research* 1:527–531.

Slack, W. V., G. P. Hicks, C. E. Reed, and L. J. Van Cura. 1966. A computer-based medical history system. *New England Journal of Medicine* 274:194–198.

Spitzer, R. L., J. Endicott, and E. Robins. 1976. Research diagnostic criteria: rationale and reliability. *Archives of General Psychiatry* 129:167–172.

Spitzer, R. L., J. Williams, M. Gibbon, and M. B. First. 1988. The Structured Clinical Interview for DSM-III-R. Biometrics Research Dept., N.Y.S. Psychiatric Institute, 722 W. 168th Street, New York City, N.Y. 10032.

Weitzel, W. D., D. W. Morgan, and T. E. Guyden. 1973. Toward a more efficient mental status examination. *Archives of General Psychiatry* 28:215–218.

5

COMPUTERIZED PSYCHOLOGICAL ASSESSMENT

Scott Wetzler

The most widespread application of computers in psychiatry and psychology has been computerized psychological assessment. Almost all psychological tests are now available in computerized format. At least two dozen companies have penetrated the psychological marketplace, offering various computerized versions of standard psychological tests. Each month the American Psychological Association *Monitor* publishes advertisements for new computer services and newly computerized tests. There is a definite market for these services, and computerized psychological assessment has become commonplace. For those companies that succeed, the revenues are impressive. While updated figures are not available, a 1985 review reported that one company alone (Psych Systems) had 320 software owners and 700 testing terminals in operation (Fowler, 1985). During the 17 years (from 1965 to 1982) that Roche Psychiatric Service Institute generated computerized MMPI reports via a mail-in service, one-fourth of the eligible psychiatrists and clinical psychologists in the United States utilized this service, for a total of 1.5 million reports.

Notwithstanding the tremendous increase and acceptance of computerized psychological assessment over the 25 years it has been available, there remain significant doubts and questions about the role of computers in psychological assessment. The intense marketing campaign conducted by these computer testing companies has essentially oversold the product. Matarazzo (1983), the most notable critic of computerized testing, refers to the "undisguised hucksterism" of these companies and to how they "tout" the tests. He predicts that computerization will lead to too much psychological testing done by ill-prepared professionals who will produce inadequate test reports. Most worrisome to Matarazzo (1983) is that the computer test report has the "spurious appearance of infallibility and objectivity" (p. 323). Not only does the computer supplant the clinician, but it appears to be a superhuman clinician. Needless to say, this claim, made implicitly or explicitly, represents a significant threat to many clinicians and confirms their worst fears of the new technology.

Based on my experience, I have found that computerization is no panacea and that it is far from flawless. Computerized test reports frequently contain gross and obvious errors of judgment as well as contradictory statements. By ignoring these weaknesses, the computer testing industry does a serious disservice to the field of psychological assessment. When used appropriately, cautiously and conservatively, however, the computer can be an important, labor-saving adjunct for the clinical psychologist conducting an assessment. It is the misuse and misapplication of computerized psychological assessment that is disappointing and irresponsible.

Everyone agrees that computers are ideally suited to certain types of psychological tests—those tests that do not require a skilled clinician for administration and scoring. Computer technology represents the most cost-effective way of administering and scoring test protocols. They are quick and objective. The controversial point, however, is whether prepackaged test interpretations are of high enough quality. Since test interpretations are often based on "actuarial" principles (Meehl, 1954), the potential of computerized psychological assessment is great. This potential has only partially been realized.

The first computerized psychological assessment services utilized the MMPI. Beginning in 1962, the Mayo Clinic in Minnesota developed a fairly simple-minded computer report that was used to screen tens of thousands of medical patients who were seen at the clinic. However, it was the national success of the Roche Laboratories' MMPI report that inspired a host of imitators and improvements. Testing services differed with regard to how they interpreted MMPI results: the nature of the underlying clinical decision rules and the library of interpretive statements. Some MMPI systems (i.e., Caldwell report) now contain as many as 30,000 interpretive sentences in their library. The next stage in the expansion of computerized psychological assessment was the introduction of different psychological tests, including other personality tests (e.g., 16-PF and Millon Clinical Multiaxial Inventory); vocational tests (e.g., Strong Campbell Interest Inventory); and tests of cognitive or intellectual ability (e.g., Wechsler Adult Intelligence Scale or Slosson Intelligence Test). Stiff competition among these companies has led to a restructuring in the industry over the last few years. Presently, there is one leading company, National Computer Systems (NCS), that dominates the field and offers a menu of several dozen psychological tests from which the user may choose.

TECHNOLOGY

Computer technology may be employed for psychological assessment in several quite different ways. The least controversial areas are administration and/or scoring of psychological tests. In each instance, the computer functions as a clerk. For test administration, the patient or client sits at a computer terminal and responds to each question displayed on the monitor. The test taker uses a keyboard, a light pencil, or a touch-sensitive screen. Computer administration significantly decreases the time required to complete a psychological test. It also appears to be a relatively pleasant experience for the subject (Johnson & Johnson, 1981). From the standpoint of test validity, one may not yet conclude with certainty whether this mode of administration influences test results in comparison to the traditional paper-and-pencil mode of administration (see Butcher et al., 1985, for a review). I suspect, however, that these two forms of test administration are equivalent when identical versions of the test are given.[1]

The greatest problem with computerized test administration is its impracticality. The patient may take as long as an hour to an hour and a half to complete an MMPI, thereby depriving others of access to the computer. Also, the clinician may be reluctant to give a psychotic patient access to such a valuable piece of machinery, although he or she would be perfectly sanguine about giving the patient a paper-and-pencil test.

Even when the computer is not used for test administration, it is extremely useful for scoring test protocols. Scoring complicated psychological tests represents the greatest benefit of computerization. Data are inputted into the computer by a clerk, who enters individual item responses, or by an optical scanner, which reads answer sheets in a second. Optical scanners designed for this purpose are affordable and very reliable. Also, the use of optical scanners for data entry dispels the possible problems associated with changing the mode of test administration, since the patient completes the test in the traditional way by paper-and-pencil.

Once the data have been entered, the computer will calculate raw scale scores and convert raw scores to standardized scores on the basis of norms. These statistical computations are done according to specific algorithms. The computer never miscounts or uses an incorrect norm, while humans do occasionally make such inadvertent errors. As these calculations become even more complex with the advent of more sophisticated psychometric tests, the need for computers will be even greater.

While most computerized psychological tests are self-report tests derived from questionnaires or inventories, there have been computerized applications of psychological tests that are administered

---

1. In my opinion, the most interesting potential "response bias" is the increased acquiescence and decreased social desirability associated with computers in comparison to paper-and-pencil administration (Jackson 1987).

by a trained clinician (e.g., Rorschach, Bender-Gestalt, or Halstead-Reitan). After the clinician administers these tests, he or she scores each response according to a standardized system, such as the Exner system for the Rorschach, and inputs these individual scores into the computer. The computer then calculates summary scores for these nonself-report tests. To my mind, such computer applications do not save much professional labor, since the clinician is still obliged to administer and score each protocol.

The most controversial aspect of computerized psychological assessment is the computer-based test interpretation (CBTI). The CBTI is a narrative report, based on test results, that resembles a typical psychological assessment report. CBTIs are generated from a library of prepackaged narrative sentences or paragraphs that describe prototypic clinical phenomena. Decision rules determine how scores are converted into narrative statements.

The CBTI represents a quantum leap in the use of computers for psychological assessment, since the computer exercises expert judgment, not merely serving as a clerk or statistician. It is the advent of the CBTI as a substitute for a live clinician that has drawn the great preponderance of criticism (Matarazzo, 1986).

COMPUTER-BASED TEST INTERPRETATIONS (CBTI)

The quality of CBTIs varies considerably from test to test and from program to program. All too often criticism of CBTIs is levied against the entire range of computer products, and weaknesses of a particular interpretive system are assumed to apply to other systems. In fact, each CBTI system is a separate entity with its own decision rules and interpretive principles.

Butcher et al. (1985) describe three basic types of CBTIs: (1) descriptive, (2) clinician modeled, and (3) clinical-actuarial. A descriptive system consists of narrative sentences that are based on individual scale scores. This analysis ignores the configuration or pattern of multiple scale scores and must therefore be simplistic. Since each individual scale is interpreted independently, the report may contain contradictory statements based on different scales.

These reports, often written in a choppy style, are an embarrassment to clinical psychology.

The clinician modeled systems are attempts to imitate the interpretive strategies of expert clinicians. How does the expert analyze test results? If his or her thought process can be made explicit, then the computer would be able to imitate it. Making certain intuitive leaps explicit is, however, a very difficult task. Needless to say, this type of CBTI is based on the assumption that the expert's interpretation is an accurate one.

The clinical-actuarial system is a mixture of a purely actuarial approach (Meehl, 1954) and the clinical approach. Tests such as the MMPI, which have been thoroughly researched, offer the opportunity to base interpretation of test profiles on empirical, systematically collected evidence. Each test profile is analyzed with regard to which scale scores are highest. Code types are defined, and have been demonstrated to be associated with certain personality features. At present, there are no purely actuarial systems because the available systems leave a significant number of patients unclassified into one or another code type. The remaining profiles must be interpreted based on clinical lore. By employing a configural or pattern recognition approach, the level of interpretation is much more complex and sophisticated; and by using an empirically derived approach, the interpretations are generally more accurate.

The debate over the quality of CBTIs is, in part, a repetition of the debate over clinical versus actuarial interpretation (Meehl, 1954). Just as clinical psychologists 30 years ago bridled at the thought that fixed interpretative rules would be an improvement over more individualized interpretative strategies, many psychologists today object to the inflexibility of computerized interpretative strategies. Given a particular code type, the computer will always make the same interpretation. The live clinician can modify his or her interpretation according to various contextual factors. Second, computers have inflexible decision rules such that a one-point differential may result in vastly different interpretations.

The quality of CBTIs depends on a number of factors, including the validity of the psychological test itself (frequently ignored in such discussions), the quality of the decision rules making up the interpretive system, and the quality and number of interpretive statements themselves. The best way to judge the accuracy and overall quality of CBTIs is to compare them to each other and to reports prepared by live clinicians (although live clinicians are by no means the gold standard). Instead, most computer test companies conduct customer satisfaction surveys that invariably reveal that the user is pleased with the product (Green, 1982). As Lanyon (1984) argues, these surveys are meaningless, since global or ambiguous interpretations may be viewed as accurate by the satisfied customer. This phenomenon is known in social psychology as the Barnum effect and may account for the popularity of astrology. More important than customer satisfaction is the discriminant validity and the incremental utility of the CBTI. Does this statement apply to this patient specifically at this point in time? And does it tell us something we did not already know?

There are several strategies for evaluating the quality of CBTIs. The primary strategy is to compare the overall report or particular statements within the report to external criteria that are rated independently. Moreland's (1985) review determined that few CBTI validation studies used adequate methodology. Even if the methodology were improved, one wonders whether the CBTI would be any less valid than the typical clinical report.[2] The second strategy for evaluating the quality of CBTIs is to evaluate the algorithms and decision rules (and associated interpretative statements) on which the CBTI is based. Since most testing companies do not permit outsiders to look at the internal structure of their programs, this strategy is for the most part unavailable.

In summary, this review reveals that CBTIs have not received adequate and sufficiently rigorous validation. It is incumbent upon the computer test industry to provide such validation. Unfortunately, their primary interest is profitability, and they seem to prefer marketing their CBTIs without such background research. Not surprisingly, many sophisticated clinicians are skeptical about these reports.

---

2. The ideological and polemical nature of the debate over CBTIs is evident when one considers that the validity of a CBTI is regularly questioned, whereas the validity of a typical clinical test report is rarely questioned and never systematically evaluated.

PROFESSIONAL ISSUES

The advent of computerized psychological assessment has presented a host of professional issues for psychologists to consider. The most important question is: Who takes clinical responsibility for the computerized test report? The computer is certainly not responsible (nor for that matter is the company that markets the test program); neither is the clerk or manager who oversees the test process. Since CBTIs are unsigned, it may appear that there is no trained professional identified as the responsible clinician. If no one does take responsibility, then psychological assessment has truly become dehumanized. The impersonal and automated context of assessment tends to encourage a lack of clarity about clinical responsibility. Responsibility is often diffused across many different figures. Herein lies the greatest danger of computerized psychological assessment: No one may take responsibility for the assessment; or alternatively, unqualified people may take responsibility and use the test findings in inappropriate ways. To make matters worse, the CBTI offers a veneer of credibility and may be more respected than a test report written by a live clinician. The layman's assumption that computers never make mistakes may cover over fundamental problems in the CBTI.

Considering the weaknesses of CBTIs and considering the opportunity for misusing them, it is particularly important that a qualified clinician review and edit all computerized test reports. A specific clinician is then responsible for the report and its repercussions. In this sense, the computerized testing program is a service to the test user (i.e., the clinician), not to the test taker. The test user can incorporate the test findings wholly, partially or not at all into his or her assessment. Matarazzo (1983) aptly compares computerized testing to the automatic pilot on an airplane: The automatic pilot is capable of flying the airplane under the constant scrutiny of the real pilot. When tricky manuevers are indicated, the real pilot will take over the controls. Similarly, while CBTIs may be able to accurately interpret uncomplicated test results, a trained clinical psychologist is needed to interpret more complicated test results and to interpret the effects of certain contextual factors on test results.

Based on these concerns, the American Psychological Association (APA) has published stringent *Guidelines for Computer-Based Tests and Interpretations* (1986). These standards define responsibilities for test users and test developers. They essentially state that users must be qualified professionals who take full clinical responsibility; and secondly, that test developers should conduct and publish extensive background research into the appropriate use of these psychological tests. The APA recommends that computer testing companies open their program to a small number of outside reviewers, to examine the CBTI decision rules that are under copyprotection.

One thorny issue that is sidestepped by the APA guidelines is the question of whether nonpsychologists are qualified to take responsibility for computerized psychological tests. While their standards are binding only to psychologists, the APA recommends that qualified nonpsychologists abide by the same principles. However, it remains an open question whether psychiatrists and psychiatric social workers have opportunities to receive adequate training in the interpretation of psychological tests. The APA merely states that all users must be fully trained and qualified.

Another important professional issue is the legal liability of test users and test developers. While there has yet to be a single lawsuit relating to a CBTI during its 25-year history, one may be certain that they will come. The courts will then determine who exactly is liable for the test findings. Legal issues surrounding privacy and confidentiality may also emerge. Finally, questions regarding billing for computerized testing will also need to be resolved. Should the clinician bill for time expended or for the service itself? If he or she bills for the service, then one may expect to see a large increase in the amount of testing conducted (considering the ease with which these tests may be administered, scored, and interpreted). Many of these issues will become clearer as computerized psychological assessment becomes a more accepted and standard practice.

A PERSONAL EXPERIENCE

My own personal experience with computerized psychological assessment may help to illustrate its strengths and weaknesses.

During the past five-and-a-half years I have headed a computerized testing program for the Department of Psychiatry at Montefiore Medical Center/Albert Einstein College of Medicine. Our program is intended to offer a standardized, quantifiable initial clinical evaluation of psychiatric patients immediately upon admission to our inpatient and outpatient psychiatric services. During this time we have assessed approximately 500 patients, which represents somewhere between 25% and 40% of all eligible patients (depending on the service and the year). To meet the needs of this clinical program, we purchased a personal computer, printer, and optical scanner, as well as the necessary testing software and test materials. The expense was minimal and the equipment is mostly used for purposes other than psychological assessment.

All psychological tests are administered by paper-and-pencil and then read by the optical scanner. On the inpatient service we offer a battery of tests, which requires two to three hours for the patient to complete at his or her leisure. In the outpatient clinic the test battery requires less than one hour to complete and is administered in weekly group testing sessions. Only the most psychotic or demented patients are unable to fill out the test materials in these structured settings. The inpatient test battery includes the Minnesota Multiphasic Personality Inventory (MMPI), the Millon Clinical Multiaxial Inventory (MCMI), and the Symptom Checklist 90 (SCL-90). The outpatient battery is limited to the MCMI and SCL-90. These tests were selected because they covered most important dimensions of psychopathology. The SCL-90 provides a profile of acute symptomatology: those problems that are currently distressing to the patient. The MCMI provides a profile of longstanding personality functioning as well as a profile of current clinical syndromes, which crossvalidates the SCL-90 findings. The MMPI is a much more cumbersome instrument to use, but its extensive history over the last 40 years makes it an excellent instrument to assess a wide range of psychopathological functions.

The computer printouts consist of raw and standardized scores on all scales, graphic presentation of these profiles, and the CBTI for the MCMI. I did not purchase CBTIs for the MMPI and SCL-90 because I was not satisfied with their quality. The final psychological assessment report is a composite of a report written by the psychologist and the CBTI. The first page is wholly written by the clinical psychologist, incorporating data from all the tests. The remainder of the report is an edited version of the CBTI from the MCMI. My own experience has been that the first section of this CBTI on longstanding personality is excellent, describing in eloquent detail the patient's basic interpersonal style; the second section on clinical syndromes is overly simplistic and gives a misleading and often inaccurate impression of diagnostic syndromes; the third section listing "noteworthy responses" is quite useful, especially in regard to self-destructive potential; the fourth section giving "suggested" *DSM-III* diagnoses is almost never correct; and the fifth section on recommended therapeutic interventions is instructive for trainees. Considering the variable quality of the CBTI, the psychologist reviews and edits it. Some sections are left intact, others are omitted entirely. The two parts of the report are then stapled together. Typically, the scoring and interpretation of these tests requires less than 20 minutes, and the report is often completed within 48–72 hours of the patient's admission.

The computerized testing program has been very favorably received by the clinical staff. The psychologists are able to consult on a large percentage of cases, and they feel that their findings are directly relevant to treatment planning. The reports are also discussed in a timely manner, that is, at the outset of the treatment planning process. While the "computerized" aspect of this assessment program gets most of the attention, I believe that the real innovation is not the technology. It is the introduction of brief, self-report tests rather than the application of more labor-intensive traditional tests, such as the Rorschach. Once we decided to use this more contemporary assessment strategy, we were then able to take advantage of the computer technology. We rely heavily on the computer and optical scanner for scoring, and we carefully and cautiously incorporate one of the CBTIs. Without the computer we would not be able to test as many patients as we do.

From the professional standpoint, the psychology staff takes full responsibility for the test report. We never allow a computerized report to be included in the chart without our review, careful editing, and signature. Based on my experience with one of the best CBTIs (i.e., the MCMI report by National Computer Systems),

I am convinced that the computerized report alone would be more misleading than beneficial. I also believe that clinical professionals who are nonpsychologists are not qualified to reinterpret the CBTI data without extensive training.

FUTURE DIRECTIONS

Computerized psychological assessment continues to have great potential. In addition to improvements in the validation of CBTIs, there are a number of other avenues for computer test development. The most promising innovation is adaptive testing, which may reduce test-taking time by 50% (Weiss, 1985). An adaptive test is tailored to the individual subject. The presentation of a new question or item is contingent upon the previous responses. Items that are determined to be irrelevant to a particular individual are omitted. Responses are related to an underlying intellectual ability or personality trait according to empirically derived probabilities. Once a psychometrically adequate estimate of this underlying dimension is obtained, no further items need to be presented. The computer can calculate these estimates instantaneously and then choose the next item to present. In essence, the computer determines a complex branching strategy. Paper-and-pencil administration does not offer this flexibility. Adaptive testing is best suited to testing intellectual abilities, where a person's baseline and ceiling may be easily and quickly determined using a predetermined sampling strategy. It may be less applicable to personality assessment, however, since the lack of homogeneity of personality dimensions makes for difficulty in determining which items have discriminatory power (Jackson, 1987).

Computer assessment also offers the opportunity to use local norms rather than standard national norms. Local norms are computed according to the local base rates (i.e., of the city, hospital, or service) and they might in fact be quite different from standard norms. Local norms would therefore improve the predictive power of the psychological test based on Bayesian mathematics. Since a computer can perform these calculations easily and would be able to constantly update the local norm, it is a necessary component of such a system.

Finally, one promising area for future development in computerized psychological testing has to do with ancillary aspects of test administration. For example, the computer can measure the individual's response time or how hard the test taker pressed the key. While these response behaviors are interesting, they may be difficult to interpret and not at all relevant. As Skinner and Pakula (1986) commented, the computer "won't tell you whether the latency was due to the client pausing to sneeze, falling off the chair, or seeing visions of Christ on the terminal" (p. 47).

In conclusion, computerized psychological assessment does have much potential. It is already very useful as a labor-saving technology. Certain CBTIs may be used in certain contexts by psychologists who have a realistic sense of the limitations. Unfortunately, the marketing of these instruments by the computer testing industry is so intense that their weaknesses are frequently overlooked. The danger that computerized test reports may be disseminated in an irresponsible way by unqualified users remains great.

REFERENCES

American Psychological Association. 1986. *Guidelines for Computer-Based Tests and Interpretations.* Washington, DC: APA.

Butcher, J. N., L. S. Keller, and S. F. Bacon. 1985. Current developments and future directions in computerized personality assessment. *Journal of Consulting and Clinical Psychology* 53:803–815.

Fowler, R. D. 1985. Landmarks in computer-assisted psychological assessment. *Journal of Consulting and Clinical Psychology* 53:748–759.

Green, C. J. 1982. The diagnostic accuracy and utility of MMPI and MCMI computer interpretive reports. *Journal of Personality Assessment* 46:359–365.

Jackson, D. N. 1987. *Computer-Based Personality Testing.* Washington, DC: APA.

Johnson, J. H. and J. N. Johnson. 1981. Psychological considerations related to the development of computerized testing stations. *Behavioral Research Methods, Instruments, and Computers* 13:421–424.

Lanyon, R. I. 1984. Personality assessment. *Annual Review of Psychology* 35:667–701.

Matarazzo, J. D. 1983. Computerized psychological testing. *Science* 221:323.

———. 1986. Computerized clinical psychological test interpretations: Unvalidated plus all mean and no sigma. *American Psychologist* 41:14–24.

Meehl, P. E. 1954. *Clinical versus Statistical Prediction: A Theoretical Analysis and a Review of the Evidence.* Minneapolis: University of Minnesota Press.

Moreland, K. L. 1985. Validation of computer-based test interpretations: Problems and prospects. *Journal of Consulting and Clinical Psychology* 53:816–825.

Skinner, H. A. and A. Pakula. 1986. Challenge of computers in psychological assessment. *Professional Psychiatry: Research and Practice* 17:44–50.

Weiss, D. J. 1985. Adaptive testing by computer. *Journal of Consulting and Clinical Psychology* 53:774–789.

6

COMPUTERS IN INTERVIEWING AND PSYCHOTHERAPY

Robert Plutchik and
Toksoz B. Karasu

At one time computers were used almost exclusively as high-speed automatic calculators. They made it possible to do statistical computations of great complexity in a very brief period, and this use of computers remains an important one. However, over the years many additional functions have been added to the repertoire of the computer. These include: natural language translation, pattern recognition, content analyses of verbal interactions, interactive teaching, and simulation. Although all of these roles of the computer have a place in psychotherapy research, the most potentially important is probably the computer as a simulator of personality, and as a simulator of the therapy interaction.

The extent to which computer models have been used in the context of psychotherapeutic interaction is not yet well known, partly because of the highly technical and specialized nature of the relevant publications and partly because of their dissemination in diverse sources, for example, engineering journals, government publications, and technical books. The fundamental basis for computer models is the rapidly developing field of artificial intelligence, but also relevant are theories of perception, cognition, learning, problem solving, psychometrics, social networks, and personality. This is clearly too much for any one individual's skills to encompass, with the result that most of the research in this field has been carried out by teams of individuals located at major university settings containing large computer systems.

In the last few years the situation has begun to change in a dramatic way due to the introduction of small but powerful microcomputers. What once required major computer installations can now, or will shortly, be duplicated on microcomputers. This possibility may lead to a revolution in psychiatric training and practice. For the first time, psychiatry has available a flexible laboratory model that can be used to create "patients" so that students at all levels may have extensive training experience with a variety of types, and with no ethical problems. The computer is tireless, and can function at any time of the day or night to provide useful educational experiences.

From another vantage point, the computer can serve in the role of interviewer of actual patients. The research to be cited in the following pages clearly indicates that computers can collect information from real people with reliability and validity, in an interesting way, and with considerable acceptance by most patients. The data can be quickly summarized and integrated and made available to the clinician in a matter of minutes.

Most controversial of all is the computer as psychotherapist. Problems here are quite formidable, yet remarkable advances have been made by the artificial intelligence community in the recognition of the meanings inherent in natural language. The simulations of the therapist are becoming increasingly more convincing, and the data already demonstrate that patients often can not distinguish computer therapists from real therapists when interacting with them by means of teletypes.

This chapter will review the literature in two general areas. The first will deal with the role of computers in psychiatric interviewing, and the second will examine the issue of the computer as a psychotherapist or as a patient.

COMPUTERS AS INTERVIEWERS

One of the earliest uses of the computer to conduct psycho-diagnostic interviews was reported by Kleinmuntz and McLean (1968). They selected samples of items from the MMPI and had 50 subjects interviewed by the computer using a computer-controlled branching system. This meant that a subset of items was given to each subject at the beginning of the testing session, and on the basis of the subject's responses to these items, certain hypotheses were formulated by the computer program regarding the specific dimensions worthy of further exploration. In practice, this implies that instead of administering all 550 MMPI items to a respondent after it has become obvious from an initial set of items that only the dimensions of schizophrenia and paranoia are relevant, the computer could branch to highly discriminating schizophrenic and paranoid items.

The results of this procedure were compared with the results of a conventionally administered MMPI. Intercorrelations between the scale scores ranged from 0 to +.94 with an average correlation of +.38. These results were encouraging but clearly suggested the need for further work. The special value of this study was that it did not simply attempt to present standard test items by computer but rather tried to approximate a clinician's directive search during interviews, and to alter the line of questioning on the basis of training, judgment and theory.

A year after this report, Stillman, Roth, Colby, and Rosenbaum (1969) described a similar computer interview called the Computer-Assisted Special Enquirer (CASE). The questions asked at any point were often contingent on the patient's previous responses, so that it was possible to go into greater depth in areas indicated as important by the patient's previous replies. Such branching instructions must be specified in advance by the person who makes up the interview. There were two kinds of questions possible. In one, the patient was presented with a multiple-choice format. In the other, he was asked to type in information (this option being useful to collect demographic information), duration of a symptom he had described earlier, and open-ended answers to special questions. Experience with CASE indicated that even severely disturbed patients were able to answer computer-presented questions without assistance. Unfortunately, no further empirical data are presented in the paper.

Maultsby and Slack in 1971 described a computer system for obtaining a psychiatric history. They described the computer as able to present questions repeatedly with varied wording before an affirmative or negative response was accepted. "Yes" answers were followed by complex groups of questions, in turn involving branching, and designed to cover each history area in depth. "No" answers resulted in instantaneous skipping of irrelevant questions.

The computer also exerted a useful control over the interviewing process. It was programmed to proceed only after an appropriate response, to reinforce the patient's progress through the interview with meaningful words of encouragement, to explain and teach the meaning of concepts not understood, and to delve further into the subject of a question whose answer was initially unknown. These factors increased the likelihood of successful completion of the interview as well as enabled the collection of standardized data both for patient care and clinical research. The computerized interview was used with 69 new admissions and was reported by therapists to be helpful in 70% of the cases.

A similar computer interview system was later described by Klein and Greist (1972). In the interview, symptoms were described and followed in two ways: Patients typed in their individual target complaints in their own words, defined complaint boundaries, and rated frequency and severity. Standardized symptom items were presented in appropriate clusters. A typed summary showed the clinician how the patients' symptoms were changing over time.

Greist and his colleagues (1973) then went on to describe a computer interview for suicide risk prediction. Twenty-two patients who had expressed suicidal ideas and 43 other nonsuicidal psychiatric patients were interviewed by computer.

The manner in which the computer branched from question to question depended on how the patient responded to each question in succession. Patients could return to earlier questions by pressing a "back" key, and could change their answers by pressing the "change" key and entering the new response. The computer determined the direction of the interview in several ways. For most questions, the patient had to answer before the next question would appear, although he could choose to skip certain particularly sensitive questions by pressing the "skip it" key. By following carefully specified branching paths, the computer asked all the appropriate questions of each person and excluded extraneous questions that would interfere with the smooth flow of the interview. The computer also had a screening mechanism that quickly terminated the interview if the patient consistently denied the existence of suicidal and/or depressive thoughts and that allowed all other patients to receive the full interview. Immediately after the interview, the computer produced a summary of the information that had been collected and four risk-state predictions.

The results of this study showed that the computer was more accurate than clinicians in predicting suicide attempts and slightly less accurate in identifying nonattempters. In terms of the patients' reactions to the interview, 52% of the suicidal patients preferred the terminal to a physician, compared to 27% of the nonsuicidal patients. Preliminary results of a related study by these authors led them to conclude that the preferences for the computer over a clinician increased as a function of the increasing social deviancy of the subject matter being described (Greist, Gustafson, Strauss, et al., 1973).

Another computer-administered interview was concerned with 193 possible life events (Schuman, Curry, Braunstein, et al., 1975). For each life event, the patient was asked to report on whether each change was small or large, good or bad, requiring help or not, and where help should come from. The computer then printed out the patients' self-weighted life events. The data revealed that the computer printout showed new problems of concern to the patient and new information on the importance of various areas. The physicians reported that communication with and management of the patient was improved in about 20% of the cases as a result of the computer interview.

A controversy exists among behavior therapists about the amount of information needed for a behavioral assessment. In order to address this issue, Angle, Ellenwood, Hay, et al. (1977) developed a computer interview that covered 26 problem areas with a pool of 3,000 questions. Most questions were presented in linear order and there was little conditional branching. Client answers indicating excess or deficit conditions were printed out.

In an effort to assess content validity, the results of interviews by clinicians were compared with computer interviews. The computer was generally found superior to human interviewers in identifying problems in the same clients. In a survey of 331 clients, the majority reported the computer interaction to be a positive experience. Most clients reported no differences in truthfulness in their response to the clinician versus the computer, and most had no objections to the computer asking personal questions.

In Scotland, an attempt was made to assess the accuracy and acceptability of computer interrogation about alcohol problems (Lucas, Mullin, Luna, & McInroy, 1977). Each of 36 patients was interviewed three times, once by the computer and once by each of two experienced psychiatrists. On most items there was no significant difference between psychiatrists and computer; however, the computer elicited significantly higher amounts of alcohol consumption than did either of the psychiatrists. In addition, 50% of the patients rated the computer interview higher than the clinician interviews and more like the "ideal medical interview."

A similar study compared manual and computer-administered versions of the Eysenck Personality Inventory on 18 psychiatric patients (Katz & Dalby, 1981). No significant differences were found between the manual and computer administrations, and an equal number of patients preferred both styles of data collection.

A number of other recent studies have been consistent with the observations reported. For example, Carr and Ghosh (1983) compared a group of phobic patients with normal volunteers on a computer interview. Although patients took much longer to complete the interviews, more than half preferred the computer, while only about 20% preferred the clinician.

These same authors (Carr, Ghosh, & Ancill, 1983) also examined the results of computer-generated interviews with clinical records for accuracy and for omissions. Forty-eight patients with complete clinical records were subsequently interviewed by computer. The interview consisted of 250 items covering personal history, health and family life. Because the computer selected further questions according to the patients' replies, less than half of the items were displayed to any one patient. Discrepancies between computer and clinician's answers were noted and an agreement score was calculated.

Agreement in individual patients ranged from 71 to 98%. Of special interest is the fact that the computer interview yielded an average of 5.4 discoveries for each patient. These included: marked concern over masturbation, criminal record, blackouts after drinking heavily, repeated firings from jobs, previous suicide attempts, recent illicit drug use, and debts. Eighty-eight percent of the patients rated the computer interview as at least as easy as talking to a clinician. Thirty-three percent of the patients found it easier to take than a conventional interview.

Consistent with these general findings is the report by Millstein and Irwin (1983) dealing with computer-acquired sexual histories in adolescent girls. The authors of this study were interested in determining the acceptability of computer interviews to adolescent patients, and to compare anxiety levels and responses to sensitive questions in adolescents interviewed by computers, by clinicians or through self-administered questionnaires.

One hundred and eight adolescent female patients were given an anxiety questionnaire, and then interviewed by either an interactive computer, a clinician, or a self-report questionnaire. Overall, the computer interview was preferred by 40% of the adolescents, the self-report questionnaire by 34% and the clinician's interview by 26%. The percentage of patients denying that they engaged in various sexual behaviors was greatest in the clinician's interviews, next for the self-report questionnaire, and relatively least for the computer interview.

These various studies that have been cited lead to a number of conclusions. Psychological assessment and interviewing by computer are now readily available to the health professions. Such assessments are reported by patients to be interesting, comfortable and private. They sometimes report greater preferences for computer interviewing than for clinician interviewing and are apparently willing to reveal more personal data and less socially desirable responses to the computer. The computer has no inhibitions about the questions to be asked of a patient and never forgets to ask anything that may be relevant. It can assign precise mathematical weights to each symptom that is elicited and make diagnostic statements on the basis of explicit rules. There is thus reason to expect an increase in the use of the computer for these functions.

COMPUTERS AS PSYCHOTHERAPISTS

As computers increased in memory and power it did not take long before researchers began to experiment with the computer as a psychotherapist. Early attempts at simulating psychotherapy were rudimentary. The main handicap was the inability of the programs to understand ordinary natural language. The first programs also lacked a conceptual base capable of modeling the patient so that rational decisions could be made about what should be said in a particular situation. Another limitation was that their output consisted of stock phrases or clumsy rearrangements of the input expressions.

The motivation to create computers as therapists was strong. Computers are economical, consistent, have a perfect memory and make no moral judgments. They can work at any time of the day or night, every month of the year, and they never tire or get bored.

Despite these obvious advantages of computers, the difficulties in creating therapy programs have been formidable. There have been three basic technical problems: (1) how to recognize natural language input; (2) how to develop a conceptual base for the program; and (3) how to construct natural language output.

Traditional grammatical methods, such as word-by-word parsing, are inadequate because of idiomatic expressions and because of the inherent ambiguity of words and phrases. The conceptual base should consist of an inference system about human nature as well as about the patient with whom the system is communicating. The generation of a natural language output requires the connection of words and phrases from lists of expressions that vary in syntax but which reflect similar meanings.

One of the earliest attempts to have the computer simulate a therapist was described by Colby, Watt, and Gilbert (1966). In their system, the input sentence was scanned for the presence of "keys";

that is, words or combinations of words such as "I" or "I love." When the program recognized any one or more of 500 keys, it triggered a response relevant to the key, and it substituted appropriate words for the response found from the input sentences. In addition, it kept statistical track of important topics so that future responses would be influenced. If input sentences did not contain keys, the program developed responses designed to steer the person away from no key topics or to return him to previous topics. The program was capable of questioning, clarifying, focusing, rephrasing and occasionally interpreting.

Eliza

The first formal model of the therapist using these ideas was called Eliza. This program contained a set of input-output rules to be used in the scanning of key words and phrases. The key words were recognized as members of a class such that all class members would generate the same response. Response sentences could consist of whole sentences or fragments. An additional feature of the input-output rules (or scripts) used in Eliza was that forced-choice "trees" could be constructed, which required subjects to chose from a limited number of alternate answers in order to continue through the tree. Entrance into a tree was determined by the subject's use of a predetermined key word. The program was expandable by the addition of key words and new input-output rules, or scripts (Quarton, McGuire, & Lorch, 1967).

In a pilot study of 24 normal subjects, Eliza was tested. A script was constructed that used sentence fragments as the basis for reply assembly when any one of 146 key words was recognized. When no key word appeared, continuatives such as "Go on, please," were employed. Nearly all the key words embedded in contexts were words commonly used to describe emotions ("hate," "love," "anger," etc.); nearly all the words in the forced-choice trees implied relationship states between individuals ("desire," "covet," etc.).

Two independent raters judged 19% of the computer responses as inappropriate according to one of the two following criteria: (1) out-of-context responses or (2) grammatically incorrect responses.

On the basis of the post-test evaluation questionnaire and interview, subjects were divided into three categories: 62% of the subjects believed that they were communicating with another human being; 21% were not certain if they were communicating with a machine or a man; 17% believed they were communicating with a machine. None of the subjects made relevant comments about the inappropriate replies, even when these were called to their attention by the investigator. Subjects became quite "involved" in the communication, independent of their beliefs.

Some of the weaknesses in Eliza are in the transformation rules. For example, the patients' response of "yes" can be transformed into any of the following four sentences:

> You seem quite positive
> You are sure
> I see
> I understand

The transformation simply ignores the message and delivers a canned reply. The program cycles through these transformations in order to provide some variety. Another problem with Eliza is that it stops its scan when it encounters a comma. Therefore, in analyzing "No, but I felt that way about my brother," it misses the main point and simply responds to the "no." In general, Eliza has difficulty with compound sentences.

Aldous

This is a highly schematic representation of some of the processes that constitute personality and their limited use in the therapeutic context (Loehlin, 1968). Aldous reacts to certain classes of inputs (e.g., men, women) with one of three emotions: fear, anger, or attraction. These emotions generate actions of withdrawal, attack, approach, conflict or indifference, and over a period of time Aldous develops both specific and general attitudes toward the objects with which he interacts.

Aldous's attitude toward any object consists of predispositions based on the three emotions (anger, fear and attraction) plus a familiarity component (a tally of his previous encounters with the object). Each of his permanent memory locations contains numbers corresponding to these four quantities. These locations in his memory are indexed by the properties that identify objects so that, given the description of an object, the attitude toward it can immediately be located. A learning subroutine develops and modifies Aldous's attitudes, depending on the outcomes of his particular encounters with his environment. Attitudes towards general classes of objects are developed as well; for example, if one of the identifying dimensions is sex, Aldous will have an attitude toward women in general as well as attitudes toward the particular women he has encountered. These generalized attitudes permit Aldous to respond sensibly to objects on his first encounter with them. Aldous also has an introspective routine that reports on the contents of his immediate memory in response to appropriate queries.

A number of interpersonal experiments were tried in which Aldous's environment consisted of another version of himself. When two strongly positive versions were interacting, the "relationship" was at first wholly positive, then occasional sequences of attack, affection and conflict occurred, and, finally, a strongly positive equilibrium was reached. The interaction of a positive and a negative model eventually reached a state of mutual hostility. Although these findings may have some implications for the process of psychotherapy, the model is relatively simple and has no language processing and limited responses.

Plato

This model of therapy assumes that all problems can be considered to be "dilemmas," and that therapy is an attempt to extricate the client from his dilemmas and to provide creative solutions (Wagman, 1980a, 1980b, 1982).

Plato contains 69 representative life-choice problems and over 400 specific and general solutions. There are 17 categories of problems related to the following areas: school issues, dating, dropping out, drugs and smoking, extracurricular activities, family relationships, financial problems, fraternity-sorority issues, interpersonal relationships, intimate relationships, living accommodations, marriage, miscellaneous, occupational choice, study habits, summer, and transfer.

The client is asked to describe the problem and then to answer a series of questions about the problem. Various solutions are proposed, which the client ranks from good to bad. Several studies with college students showed that students who worked with Plato showed a significantly greater improvement in their problems as compared to the control group. This improvement was sustained over a one-month follow-up; it was also found that many students preferred working with the computer to seeing a counselor.

These various examples that have been given—of Eliza, Aldous, and Plato—represent ways that the computer has been programmed to take the role of a psychotherapist. This is not the only way the computer can be used in a psychotherapy context. It can also be programmed to take the role of a patient. Such use of the computer has important implications for the training of psychotherapists; it also contributes to the theoretical understanding of psychopathology. Three examples will be given here: the computer as an anxious patient, a paranoid patient, and a schizophrenic patient.

COMPUTERS AS PATIENTS

The Computer as an Anxious Patient

In this study, Colby (1964) used the experiences of a particular woman patient who was anxious and indecisive in her relations to men as the basis for his model. In the simple English that the system uses there are only nouns and verbs, although modifiers can determine the tense. A dictionary contains all the words (257) that are to appear in output sentences. Each term is part of a broader class and may also have illustrations. The program also contains 105 beliefs; that is, propositions assumed to be true.

The program searches for conflicts in the belief system. When it is found, anxiety is raised. As the model was activated four properties were observed: (1) it had a high level of anxiety (conflict);

(2) it had repeated anxiety attacks; (3) its behavior became stereotyped over time; and (4) its information output contained many contradictions. Colby found this demonstration helpful in understanding the patient.

The Computer as a Paranoid Patient

Some years later Colby developed a more sophisticated model of a paranoid patient (Colby, 1976, 1981). In this model, paranoid responses are a function of external input and current internal states. A major preoccupation of the paranoid individual is a constant searching for evidence of inadequacy of the self, which, if found, leads to the emotion of shame. Anticipation of humiliation leads to the transfer of blame to other people.

The actual model used a large concept dictionary to recognize natural language input and to match the incoming concept name to stored patterns in the model's memory. Other processes in the program involved a belief system (about self, the interviewer and the setting), ways to change the belief system, and ways to deal with affects, intentions, and actions. The model was capable of three affects: fear, anger, and shame. When the shame was raised above a critical threshold, the paranoid mode switched on, which led to certain paranoid beliefs as well as to intentions to attack the interviewer (Colby, 1976).

In a follow-up of this model (PARRY 2), Faught, Colby, and Parkison (1977) describe the dictionary as containing 1,900 entries and 500 patterns. Each affect that is recognized is stored as a number. The 50 beliefs in the system refer to topic areas that can conceivably change in the course of one interview, such things as beliefs about the self or about the interviewer. The inference mode contains 150 rules of inference, that is, rules that enable new conclusions to be drawn about new situations. Goals are designed to satisfy affects. The model contains 12 intentions; that is, linguistic action patterns capable of satisfying needs of the system or reducing the intensity of affects. Examples are: insults, lying, withdrawal, praise, information seeking, and changing the subject. Affects are assumed to weaken gradually over time.

Having developed the computer model of a paranoid patient, Heiser, Colby, Faught, and Parkison (1979) then went on to determine whether psychiatrists, using a teletype mediated interview, could distinguish a computer model of paranoia from a paranoid person. Five psychiatrists agreed to interview, via a teletype machine, a real patient, a computer, or both. After each interview the judges were asked to decide how certain they were of whether they were interviewing a computer or a patient.

The real patient was a 22-year-old male inpatient suffering from severe paranoid thinking. The computer program was a model of a 28-year-old-male inpatient with various delusions of persecution (PARRY 2). The results showed that the judges were correct five times and wrong five times, a random result. This implies either that the computer program is a good model of paranoia or that the judges are poor. The advantage of having the model is that it provides a useful laboratory experience for students, and one that enables students to learn and practice a complex skill.

In his latest version of PARRY, Colby (1981) describes the general process of modeling. First, he distinguishes between paranoid schizophrenia, which his model is not, and paranoia, which is a way of thinking or strategy that attempts to minimize or forestall shame-induced distress.

The computer model begins with a general-purpose "parser." This module takes a linear sequence of words as input and produces a treelike structure of nested phrases. These are matched to abstract rules using a conceptual thesaurus of 4,500 word stems that define general concept patterns, of which there are about 2,000. All the data tables are stored as lists.

In the model, the strength of each affect is represented by a numerical value ranging from 0 to 10. The intensity decays over time by a fixed amount. The model also contains 80 beliefs that are potentially changeable during the course of a single interview. In addition it has 130 rules of inference and 1,800 output utterances classified by meaning of a concept. Although the number of possible actions has been decided in advance, the specific action selected is decided by the system itself depending on the nature of the input and internal states.

The model of PARRY is probably the most sophisticated computer simulation extant and is still undergoing modification.

The Computer as a Schizophrenic Patient

CHRIS is a simulation of an initial diagnostic interview of a patient with an undifferentiated schizophrenic disorder. Upon completion of the interview, a teacher function of the program asks the user to indicate: (1) the types of symptoms she/he thinks the simulation displayed; (2) a diagnosis based on the interview; and (3) the rationale for that diagnosis. The program checks the user's diagnosis for accuracy; it reports a corrected diagnosis if necessary; and, finally, it lists all schizophrenic symptoms displayed during that interview. Symptoms in the program that were not encountered during the interview are also available to the user.

During the interview CHRIS is able to give up to 40 different responses that are associated with schizophrenia. The program also contains 160 responses describing its demographic background. If the input sentence contains words unknown to the program, the model will use an alternate output strategy. This includes: changing the subject, asking a question, or giving a noncommital response. The model includes about 800 words with their parts of speech, about 150 links to connect identified key phrases with output sentences and about 200 canned output responses. Interesting as this program is, it has had limited use.

SOME THEORETICAL DEVELOPMENTS

A number of researchers have developed models of memory, meaning, and social interaction. These models are important because they express psychological theories and indirectly test them. The construction of a computer model helps make the theory more precise and requires an explicit statement of all assumptions. Two examples will be given.

Malone (1975) has developed a program called DYAD, which is based on Leary's personality theory. This theory assumes that 16 basic dimensions arranged in a circle, or circumplex, can be used to describe the personality profile of any individual. In the computer model, each person's role is described in terms of a probability distribution over the 16 personality dimensions; that is, at any given time, there is a certain likelihood that an individual will act assertively, competitively, dominatingly, or passively. These probabilities change as a function of the behavior of the other person on each of the 16 dimensions. The model assumes that the probability of a response in a given category increases if it is positively reinforced, decreases if it is negatively reinforced, and is also influenced by the rate of positive or negative reinforcement.

These assumptions were programed into the computer model and two-person interactions were simulated. Consistent with Leary's theory, one of the results obtained was that people tend to provoke each other to increasing repetition of responses characteristic of each of their roles. It was also found that the rate of positive or negative reinforcement had a large effect on changes in the personality role distributions.

Four hypothetical psychiatric patients were described: (1) sadistic-aggressive; (2) masochistic; (3) paranoid, rebellious; and (4) "normal," with equal probability of response in each of the 16 categories. As these hypothetical people interacted, several results were observed. When a normal person interacted with an abnormal one, the abnormal one usually stayed the same, and the normal person changed in such a way as to elicit the characteristic responses of the other role. When one person was programmed to act as a "therapist" and to give consistently loving responses, this did not reinforce the abnormalities, but tended to change the abnormal individuals into loving ones. The model thus has value in testing hypotheses about psychotherapeutic and other types of human interactions.

Another important theoretical development that is relevant to psychotherapy simulation is the work of the artificial intelligence community, as represented, for example, by Schenk (1977) and by Lehnert (1978). These researchers have been concerned with modeling knowledge structures such as cognitions, memory and goals.

A brief description of the work of Lehnert will illustrate these ideas.

One of the major problems for the adequate modeling of psychotherapy concerns the issue of understanding English language input. How can it be demonstrated that a person or a computer "understands" a story? Lehnert suggests 16 principles that relate to the understanding of questions. They include such ideas as: questions are understood on many levels; the more inferences an answer carries, the better the answer; the same question does not always get the same answer; and a good strategy knows when it has the answer and can stop asking questions.

The primary idea underlying this question-answering model, called QUALM, is a theory of memory which assumes that the meaning of a sentence can be decomposed into a small set of primitive actions. These actions are: the transfer of physical location; the transfer of possession or control; the application of a physical force; the transfer of information; the internalization of an external object into an animal's system; the act of pushing an object out of the body; the movement of an animal; any vocal act; the focusing of a sense organ toward some stimulus; and the act of securing contact with an object. Interestingly, four of these primitive acts correspond to Plutchik's basic or prototype emotion dimensions (Plutchik, 1980).

These meanings are related in the computer model to "scripts" and "plans." Scripts are memory units containing information about frequently encountered situations. They describe the general expectations involved in such simple activities as shopping, driving, eating, and so forth. Plans are used when scripts do not apply or when they contain insufficient information. The same plan can be used in a variety of settings; for example, getting information from the library, or using a map, or buying a stock. Plans that are frequently used may eventually create scripts.

The process of finding and formulating an answer involves two basic processes: content specification and memory search. These in turn require four levels of interpretation: (1) conceptual parse, (2) memory internalization, (3) conceptual categorization, and (4) inferential analysis. In the same way that a set of primitive acts is used for the representation of acts, a set of primitive objects is used to represent physical objects (or nouns).

Although this research and computer model is not used directly for psychotherapeutic dialogue, the general theory and techniques developed to deal with question-answering dialogues will undoubtedly have relevance to therapeutic conversation.

CONCLUSIONS AND IMPLICATIONS

This review has attempted to provide an historical perspective on the use of computers in psychiatry. Over the past 20 years or so there has been an increasing use of computers in two contexts: as a clinically appropriate and flexible interviewer of patients; and as a simulator of either the therapist or the patient.

The literature reveals that the first task can be successfully accomplished by computers. A series of papers are described that clearly demonstrate that computers can present questions to patients in a clinical way, and that patients find the interactions acceptable. In fact, the data show that a sizable proportion of the patients prefer the computer interview to one with a real clinician. The results also indicate that patients tend to reveal more personal and embarrassing things to the computer then to the clinician. In the light of such findings, it seems likely that the role of the computer as interviewer will expand.

The place of the computer in psychiatry and psychology as a psychotherapist or as a patient is more problematical. A few demonstrations have been provided by a small number of investigators that a computer can be programmed to act somewhat like a therapist. But all such demonstrations have been done over very brief periods measured in minutes. How the computer-therapist will fare over sessions is simply unknown. That the therapist can simulate a patient has also been demonstrated in at least two cases, and the simulations have been real enough to sometimes fool clinicians. Here, too, the patient has been exposed only to the clinicians for a single session, and it is not known what would happen after repeated interviews.

These results are not overwhelming when one considers the advances that have been made in computer technology. What once required large mainframe computers and exotic programming languages can now be duplicated on powerful microcomputers that anyone can own. Advances in this field will probably depend on a large number of interested individuals having access to such computers with the help of skilled programmers. However, one of the key elements needed for the development of this field is an explicit theory of therapy. Unless the postulates and rules of interaction of a given form of therapy are made explicit, the programmers will be unable to do their job. The other key element needed for advance is the development of computer models of the mind so that computers can understand linguistic input in ways that are similar to the ways that humans understand it. Only after the technical aspects of language understanding are dealt with will it be possible to explore the nature of computer-human relationships in a systematic way. The prospects are exciting, but there is much yet to be done.

REFERENCES

Angle, H. V., E. H. Ellenwood, W. M. Hay, T. Johnsen, L. R. Hay. 1977. Instrumentation and techniques: computer-aided interviewing in comprehensive behavioral assessment. *Behavior Therapy* 8:747–754.

Carr, A. C., A. Ghosh, and R. J. Ancill. 1983. Can a computer take a psychiatric history? *Psychological Medicine* 13:151–158.

Carr, A. C., and A. Ghosh. 1983. Response of phobic patients to direct computer assessment. *British Journal of Psychiatry* 142:60–65.

Colby, K. M. 1964. Experimental treatment of neurotic computer programs. *Archives of General Psychiatry* 10:220–227.

———. 1976. Clinical implications of a simulation model of paranoid processes. *Archives of General Psychiatry* 33:854–857.

———. 1981. Modeling a paranoid mind. *The Behavioral and Brain Sciences* 44:515–534.

Colby, K. M., J. B. Watt, and J. P. Gilbert. 1966. A computer method of psychotherapy: preliminary communication. *The Journal of Nervous and Mental Disease* 142:148–152.

Faught, W. S., K. M. Colby, and R. C. Parkison. 1977. Inferences, affects, and intentions in a model of paranoia. *Cognitive Psychology* 9:153–187.

Greist, J. H., D. H. Gustafson, F. F. Strauss, G. L. Rowse, T. P. Laughren, and J. A. Chiles. 1973. A computer interview for suicide-risk prediction. *American Journal of Psychiatry* 130:1327–1332.

———. Suicide risk prediction: a new approach. *Life Threatening Behavior* 4:212–223.

Heiser, J. F., K. M. Colby, W. S. Faught, and R. C. Parkison. 1979. Can psychiatrists distinguish a computer simulation of paranoia from the real thing?: The limitations of Turing-like tests as measures of the adequacy of simulations. *Journal of Psychiatric Research* 15:149–162.

Katz, L., and T. Dalby. 1981. Computer and manual administration of the Eysenck Personality Inventory. *Journal of Clinical Psychology* 37:586–588.

Klein, M. H., and J. H. Greist. 1972. History of computerized psychiatric history-taking. *Journal of the American Medical Association* 220:1246–1247.

Kleinmuntz, B., and R. S. McClean. 1968. Computers in behavioral science: diagnostic interviewing by digital computer. *Behavioral Science* 13:75–80.

Lehnert, W. G. 1978. *The process of question answering: a computer simulation of cognition.* Hillsdale, NJ: Lawrence Erlbaum.

Loehlin, J. C. 1968. Machines with personality. *Science Journal* 4:97–101.

Lucas, R. W., P. J. Mullin, C. B. X. Luna, and D. C. McInroy. 1977. Psychiatrists and a computer as interrogators of patients with alcohol-related illnesses: a comparison. *British Journal of Psychiatry* 131:160–167.

Malone, T. W. 1975. System simulation: computer simulation of two-person interactions. *Behavioral Science* 20:260–267.

Maultsby, M. C., Jr., and W. V. Slack. 1971. A computer-based psychiatry history system. *Archives of General Psychiatry* 5:570–572.

McGuire, M. T., S. Lorch, and G. C. Quarton. 1967. Man-machine natural language exchanges based on selected features of unrestricted input, II. The use of the time-shared computer as a research tool in studying dyadic communication. *Journal of Psychiatric Research* 5:179–191.

Millstein, S. G., and C. E. Irwin, Jr. 1983. Acceptability of computer-acquired sexual histories in adolescent girls. *Journal of Pediatrics* 103:815–819.

Plutchik, R. 1980. *Emotion: A psychoevolutionary synthesis.* New York: Harper and Row.

Quarton, G. C., M. T. McGuire, and S. Lorch. 1967. Man-machine natural language exchanges based on selected features of unrestricted input, I. The development of time-shared computers as a research tool in studying dyadic communication. *Journal of Psychiatric Research* 5:165–177.

Santo, Y., and A. Finkel. 1982. "Chris": A computer simulation of schizophrenia. *Proceedings of the 6th Annual Synposium on Computer Applications in Medical Care* October: 737–741.

Schenk, R. C. 1977. *Scripts, plans, goals and understanding: An inquiry into human knowledge structures.* Hillsdale, NJ: Lawrence Erlbaum.

Schuman, S. H., H. B. Curry, M. L. Braunstein, R. Schneeweiss, G. C. Jebaily, N. M. Glazer, J. R. Cahn, and W. H. Crigler. 1975. A computer administered interview on life events: improving patient-doctor communication. *The Journal of Family Practice* 2:263–269.

Stillman, R., W. T. Roth, K. M. Colby, and C. P. Rosenbaum. 1969. An on-line computer system for initial psychiatric inventory. *American Journal of Psychiatry* 125:8–11.

Wagner, M. 1980a. Plato DCS: An interactive computer system for personal counseling. *Journal of Counseling Psychology* 27:16–30.

———. 1980b. Plato DCS: An interactive computer system for personal counseling: Further development and evaluation. *Journal of Counseling Psychology* 27:31–39.

———. 1982. Solving dilemmas by computer or counselor. *Psychological Reports* 50:127–135.

PART III

ESTABLISHMENT OF DATABASES IN MENTAL HEALTH SYSTEMS

7

RUDIMENTS FOR ESTABLISHING DATABASES IN MENTAL HEALTH SYSTEMS

Robert S. Kennedy

We expect as much from our machines as we expect from ourselves; sometimes we are pleased, sometimes we are disappointed.

We live in a world where rapid access to information is so much a part of our lives that it has become a necessity. Computers have made this availability and management of data possible in everything from obtaining a balance at a bank to shopping with a credit card. So, too, the health and mental health fields have seen the need for a more sophisticated system of managing the information that is used every day. It is with this as our new mandate that we cross into the age of the computer.

There are a variety of uses for a computer in any institution or office setting. For purposes of this discussion, I will focus only on utilizing a database to manage patient information.

SETTING UP A DATABASE FOR PATIENT MANAGEMENT

What most people do not realize is that when you wish to set up a database for anything, you have to know very well what you want to include in that database and what you intend to do with it.

Someone who just wants a name, address and phone list has a relatively simple job. Databases are great for a Rolodex-type file, and these are easy to construct. The difficulty comes into play when you are unsure of what to put into the database.

Think About the Data

It is wise to spend some time before you approach the computer sitting with a piece of paper and a pencil. List the items that you absolutely need to collect first, then list the less important items and so on. Be aware that when you show this list to someone else and ask them for a consultation, they will inadvertently add more items while you are trying your best to keep this list small.

Remember, the more you collect, the more space it takes up. In computer technology terms, space costs money.

What to Collect

Every day we use a variety of forms that we fill out to provide us with reference information on patients. We may wish to obtain a patient's name, mailing address, or telephone number. We might want to access a patient's diagnosis or to know when the last treatment plan was completed.

In the noncomputer world, we look at a patient's chart for this information or we keep an alphabetized card file that offers us quick reference in a small three-by-five box.

But what if we need more information on many patients? We can buy a bigger box and more cards! Now, what if you need to know how many patients are under a particular age and with a particular diagnosis? Suddenly, you are spending a great deal of time counting and sifting through your cards. As the requests become more complex, so does the method of obtaining that information. The time to search for all these facts also becomes extended.

Now It Is Time to Bring in the Computer!

Imagine having the ability to access information in very short periods of time: that report to remind you to update a portion of your chart; that list of patients by age or diagnosis or type of medication or date of last physical exam.

A database is like a card file that allows speedy access to all the cards you need for the information you want without having to look at each card for that information.

Set Up the Database

Another way to visualize a database is to view it as a file folder in which you want to place facts organized in a particular way. Part of the design of the database is to figure out what facts you want to collect. A simple example is a database as a phone/address book. Here you would collect names, addresses, telephone numbers, and maybe birthdays.

Each of these items is called a "field." A database is composed of a number of fields. The number of fields you have in a database is generally up to you. Many people who set up databases separate specific fields, such as last name, first name, street address, city, state, zip code. This is done to make the process of retrieving the information more specific and faster. For example, you might want a list of people organized by zip code for mailing purposes or for a demographic study. It is far easier to create a separate field for the zip code than it is to search the contents of an address field for the occurrence of a particular zip code. Databases are designed for rapid searches *if* you follow the rules of the database.

The computer is extremely concrete. It cannot anticipate your needs and it gives you only what you ask for. If you make a typographic error, it reads your request literally. It does not look for a close match to anticipate what you wanted. It looks for what you asked for only.

Databases are frequently obstinate as well, to the point of being particular about capitalization. If you ask the database to find SMITH (all caps) but it is written in the database *name field* as Smith (initial cap with the rest lower case), it will report to you that it is *not* there! If you think about it . . . it isn't, at least not the way you asked for it.

Sample Database Setup

Field	Size	Type of Field
Last Name	25	Character
First Name	15	Character
Street Address	30	Character
City	15	Character
State	2	Character
Zip Code	5	Character
Birth Date	8	Date
Balance	7	Numeric

What does all this mean?

A *field,* as described above, is one of the items in the database. The *size* is the number of spaces that you determine this field requires (maximum length) and the *type* of field is a way of telling the database how to store the data and how the information will be utilized. There are different field types: character fields; numeric fields; date fields; or logic fields; each with a specific purpose.

All of these together constitute a *record.* A record is analogous to a file or card on someone.

When you input information into the database, you will be filling in the blank fields. It probably would look something like this:

Record   1

LASTNAME	[SMITH]
FIRSTNAME	[CHARLES]
ADDRESS	[1234 SMITHTOWN ROAD]
CITY	[QUEENS]
STATE	[NY]
ZIP	[10010]
BIRTHDATE	[01/02/60]
BALANCE	[25.00]

As mentioned earlier, defining the database requires some structuring of the information before you even sit down at the computer. You need to carefully prepare for the way the information will be put in. It is far more difficult later to go back and change your mind after you have typed in 200 names and addresses.

Other types of fields that are useful for collection of general information are:

Sex
Ethnicity
Marital status
Admission date
Readmission date
Family income
Number of people in household
Work phone
Family or friend to contact in case of emergency
Patient case number
Social security number

General information can easily be combined with billing information to facilitate management and billing by adding fields such as:

Fee
Insurance carrier and number
Medicaid or medicare number or both

Last visit
Number of visits this month

Clinical Data

After deciding what *general* background information to collect, the next task is to assess what *clinical* information you wish to put into the database.

To avoid the pitfalls of putting too much information or unnecessary data into the database, the point here is to think about the end result of the information. When deciding what to collect, you need to assess what you are going to do with the information. The *end result* of data collection is a report of some kind. *Reports* are designed to organize the data from the database and present it in some organized way to the reader to communicate specific information. Reports will be discussed later.

One clinical entity that most clinicians deem crucial is a diagnosis. The consideration here is whether to put the information in numeric form or in descriptive form. For example, you could create a diagnosis field that contains either the written-out diagnosis, such as dysthymic disorder or the code 300.40. Both ways are useful; it depends on what your needs are. If you are more concerned with creating a medicaid or medicare bill, the numeric is more important. If you want to create a report that lists a patient, mailing address, therapist's name, and diagnosis, you might wish to see the diagnosis spelled out rather than decipher a list of numbers.

Again, the consistency of entering the information is crucial. If you are creating a special list by diagnosis or counting the number of schizophrenic patients you have on your service, misspelled diagnoses or typographical errors will be overlooked and thus not counted, whereas coded entries are less prone to mistakes.

Other fields that might be clinically useful to include when constructing your database are:

Date of last treatment plan review
Axis 2, 3, 4 and 5 diagnoses

Estimated level of functioning (use or set up a scale)
History of previous suicide attempts
History of previous violent acts
Family history of emotional disorders or alcoholism
Previous psychiatric history or hospitalizations
Psychiatric medications
Date of last prescription (refills?)
Nonpsychiatric medications
Name and number of family doctor
Medical problems
Allergies
Evidence of tardive dyskinesia (via a scale)
Last prescription date
Date of last physical exam
Number of siblings or names
Parents' names
Education or grade completed

Fields intended for billing or demographics can also benefit the clinician. Showing the admission date or calculating the length of treatment might be useful, as well as showing age or sex statistics, ethnic characteristics, and so forth.

Space Considerations

Before we make the database too large, space—the amount of storage that a database utilizes—needs to be considered. The above database (composed of first name, last name, address, city, zip, birthdate, and balance) could hold approximately 3,500 records before filling a 5.25″ floppy disk on an IBM PC or compatible computer.

Integrity of Data

Inputting information or entering data needs to be as consistent as possible. As mentioned above, the computer is concrete. A good rule of thumb is to keep or enter all information in all capital letters; otherwise you will have serious problems in retrieving the information. This is especially important to watch if you have more than one person entering the data.

THE COMPUTER-TO-HUMAN INTERFACE

The Human Interface Must Be as Easy as Possible

Another crucial element in managing patient data with a computer system is *not* the computer system but the "computer-to-human interface." Frequently, this requires the savvy and sophistication of a skilled psychotherapist. Staff have two initial reactions to a computer: first, they are intimidated and overwhelmed; and second, they expect too much. What the average person sees on television is not what you are going to show them or do for them. No flash. No fancy colors. No rotating graphics. When they get past the fear of "What if I push the wrong button, will I wipe out everything?" they will be impressed with the technology and disappointed with the plain businesslike screens.

The best approach to minimizing the resistant or intimidated staff is to *make everything possible menu driven. Menu driven* means that when the computer is turned on, a menu or list of choices appears and you are simply required to push a button corresponding to your choice. A simple example would look like this:

```
*  = = = = = = = = = = = = = = = *
*        Patient Database System         *
*                                        *
*                Main Menu                *
*        _____              *
*        I.  Enter new information        *
*                                         *
*        2,  Edit current information     *
*                                         *
*        3.  Printed Reports              *
*                                         *
*        4.  Quit                         *
*                                         *
*  = = = = = = = = = = = = = = = *
```

Keeping the choices as simple and as minimally confusing as possible helps make a system work with little effort and few mistakes.

A frequent topic in discussions of clinical charting is *progress notes*. Writing chart notes to keep in a computer is being tried in many institutions. Again, the issues here are twofold: (1) Who is going to put in the information? and (2) How much storage space do you have?

Unless you equip each clinician with a computer and train him or her to use your particular program, it is going to be difficult to get daily chart notes put in a computer. This is probably what will occur 10 years from now. A small computer on everyone's desk will be as necessary as the telephone for our daily lives; but, for now, it is a problem of equipment costs and training. Do you have a secretary type in your clinical notes? You then have to assess for the consistency and integrity of the data being typed in.

Space again is a serious consideration. Notes take up much more space than a simple database. Like office space, no matter how much you plan ahead, you will be looking to stretch the space you have.

The Paperless Office

The paperless office is one of the great myths of our time. If anything, the computer generates more paper. It produces not only information faster but also more reports faster than before.

Now everyone wants a report!

The last element of the computer-to-human interface that we will discuss is the *report*.

Who Gets the Information and Who Needs It?

The people who should benefit the most from information collected by a computer system are the people who can make the most use of the information. Contrary to popular convention, it should not be the MIS managers or administrators. In a clinical setting, the clinician should benefit from the most immediate results of computer information. Of course, the management staff needs to view and assess the range of diagnoses or geographic location of a particular set of patients; but it is just as important to a clinician to have ready access to patient telephone numbers, due dates of treatment plan reviews, and clinical problems on his/her particular patient caseload.

A clinician who completes daily activity reports or patient contact reports should have at *least* a monthly report from all of his or her efforts.

Reports in a database system can be kept relatively simple and should be very easy to read. A report full of lots of numbers or statistical formulas instantly loses the reader and confuses most people.

A sample report could read:

01/01/88
Active Caseload
Report for Staff => John Jones

Patient	Chart #	Last Visit	Number of Visits in last 3 months
John Smith	1111111	12/01/87	12
Address			
City, State Zip			
Phone			
*			
Alfred Smith	2222222	10/12/87	5
Address			
City, State Zip			
Phone			
*			

Graphics are a clever way to inform or communicate information. A simple example would be:

01/01/88
Group Therapy—Tuesday 10 A.M. Group
Report for Staff => John Jones

Patient	Chart #	Visits for First Half of 1987						
		1	5	10	15	20	25	30
John Smith	1111111	* *						
Alfred Smith	2222222	* * * * * * * * *						
Peter Edwards	3333333	* * * * * * * * * * * * *						
Susan Peterson	4444444	* *						

Another variation would be:

	Jan	Feb	Mar	Apr	May	June
Smith	2	4	1	6	4	8
Jones	2	6	4	2	2	7
Rivera	3	3	3	4	3	3
Connors	4	4	4	4	2	2
Lee	1	2	1	3	4	1
Majors	2	2	2	1	2	2
Romero	4	4	2	4	4	2
Jackson	1	4	8	2	3	1

Patient visits for first 6 months

Reports can convey various kinds of information and they can be modified for different readers. Managers will be interested in one type of report, while a clinician will look for other types of data on their patients.

For the most part, reports are the bottom line or the end result of a patient database. If any one issue determines the average person's impression of the value of computer information more than most other aspects, the report is what is most visible and most sought after.

WHAT DOES A COMPUTER DATABASE
FOR PATIENT MANAGEMENT OFFER?

1. *Concentration of information (availability) and speed of access.*
Because the information is concentrated in one place and organized, access is quick and accurate.

2. *Flexibility of ways to view data.*
Information can be viewed or asked for in a variety of ways. It can be presented in reports or graphs or combined in unique ways.

3. *Clinical directions for patient management or training; i.e., the ability to assess diagnostic directions and direct training toward shifts in population, etc.*

Examples:
A clinic can assess how many single mothers on public assistance are in the clinic and whether a support group for the mothers and a prevention group for the children should be started.

Should a geriatric group be organized now that the data shows that the over-sixty population is increasing?

Recently, caseloads have been shown to have a large number of substance abusers. Should more staff training be instituted?

4. *Administrative directions for hiring.*

Example:
Data can show if there is a need to hire a bilingual therapist.

5. *Flow control and productivity.*

Examples:
Highs or lows in monthly statistics can be viewed along with statistics for each clinician.

An overview of contents of a particular therapist's caseload can be seen.

A direction for what kinds of groups are needed can be shown.

Average length of treatment or number of readmissions each year can be tracked.

There are also specific types of clinical information that can be obtained.

1. *Diagnostic information.*
General as well as specific diagnostic information can be outlined.

2. *Treatment plans.*
Patient strengths and problems can be listed and quickly recalled.

Date of treatment plan information can signal due dates of treatment plan reviews.

Special problems can be flagged to assess progress or change.

3. *Treatment plan reviews.*
Dates from the treatment plan can signal when a review is due.

Problems from the treatment plan can be recalled and assessed for change.

4. *Patient self-assessment.*
It is even possible to have a patient fill out his or her own treatment plan and keep a log of changes.

5. *Level of functioning information over time.*
Changes can be recorded. This can also be part of a treatment plan review or a separate scale.

In an outpatient day program setting or day hospital, functioning scales can be logged daily or weekly. Goals can be established and progress can be graphed.

6. *Medication follow-up.*
Using fields such as date of last prescription and amounts prescribed, the computer can tell you when a patient is due for a refill and make inferences as to whether a patient is taking his/her medication properly.

7. *Caseload management.*

Date of last visit or next visit can help a clinician manage his or her caseload and pick up on those patients who do not follow through well or who "fall through the cracks" in a mental health system.

8. *Alert fields.*

If a patient is checked as suicidal, a therapist can be notified quickly if the last appointment was missed.

These are just some of the possibilities. The list is as endless as our ability to create and solve problems.

SUMMARY

Provided sufficient time is given to intelligent planning, a database for patient management can be a viable tool in a mental health setting. We need new ways to view what we do. We need new ways to synthesize the volumes of information that we collect every day. We need, most of all, new ways to interface all of this new technology to broaden our perspective without losing sight of why we are here.

8

INTEGRATED DATABASES FOR CLINICAL CARE AND RESEARCH IN PSYCHOPHARMACOLOGY

David Gastfriend

Computer database technology has not caught on in medicine and psychiatry at the rate we might have expected. To a large extent it has remained a disappointment to medical and psychiatric users. For over a decade it has been well known that computerized databases are efficient and cost-effective tools in business and scientific applications. In our fields their use has lagged, partly because of the difficulty in capturing the richness of the medical record and because of a lack of sufficiently easy-to-use software for nonprogrammers. Clinicians have been especially unable to appreciate what database management systems are.

It is not surprising that many proponents of this technology have become disappointed at the slow pace of acceptance of database technology in medicine. In 1969, Octo Barnett, Director of the Laboratory of Computer Science at the Massachusetts General Hospital, asked, "What is the cause of this state of underachievement?" In 1977, a survey of computerized medicine systems found that only 19% were still being routinely used (Friedman & Gustafson, 1977). By 1981, a study of 22 active computerized hospital information systems revealed the discouraging finding that only 20% of admitting doctors made any use of them (Young, 1984).

When Barnett (1986) reviewed the status of clinical information systems in the *New England Journal of Medicine,* a letter to the editor critically responded, "There has been little implementation of computer-based medical record systems by an American medical community with an avidity for new technology. Why has there not been progress? Because there is inadequate evidence that computerized records lead to better medical and economic outcomes, and anyway, the record is self serving . . . selective, defensive and biased" (Anderson, 1984). Barnett agreed with that statement but held that these charges constituted an argument *for* the introduction of computer systems, with their potential to stimulate completeness and to make the medical record more accessible, better organized, and more easily monitored. I would add that for psychiatry, computers have the potential to make the clinical record more reliable, for example, more similar between different clinicians. Barnett (1984a) wrote that the slower-than-expected adoption of the computerized approach is due to the lack of appreciation of the complexities involved in the development and dissemination of computer-based medical record systems.

THE DATABASE CONCEPT: DATA AND FILES

The following is a brief, concrete discussion of the concept of a database management system. Consider the nature of an item "1.3." Is it data or a label? It is not a label, but if one gives it a label, for example, milliequivalents per litre, then 1.3 meq/L is an element of data, representing the value of a patient's lithium level. The lithium level is something that would vary from patient to patient, or from lab test to lab test, so that lithium level is the variable, 1.3 is the value, milliequivalents per litre is the label, and 1.3 milliequivalents per litre is now an element of data. It is still not information, however, because information is data that has been processed and helps us make a decision. If we know that this is a particular patient's lithium level at a given dose, then 1.3 milliequivalents per litre becomes information toward making a treatment decision.

Data may consist of numbers, codes, alphabetical characters, abbreviations, or whole words. Free text (or English-language) entries, a narrative statement of a patient's history of present illness, or even a whole paragraph can be data. A formula, such as a quadratic equation, can be data. Drawings, x-rays, and photographs of patients can be data. For $500 one can attach to the printer print-head a tiny camera that digitizes any picture inserted in the carriage, and store the data in a database for graphic images.

The design of any computerized database management system begins by listing the data one wants to store. One may ask, What data are we currently gathering on paper—let's make that the data we are going to store. It is even better to ask, What information do we really need to make our treatment decisions? This step is called systems analysis, and it is the most important part of developing the database. Most importantly, database systems analysis should not be conducted by a programmer or by a computer "hacker," but rather by the person who is going to use the information—the clinician. Thus it is essential that clinicians understand why the database can be helpful. In the best of all possible worlds that database should be so easy to use that the clinician should be able to modify it. Wiederhold (1981) has written a good introductory paperback for using medical databases.

The simplest kind of database is a file management system, like a file-card box for references or a Rolodex device for telephone numbers. Another file management system is the patient's visit note, where the note is written on a piece of paper placed in the chart, which in turn is stored in a Pendaflex folder in a particular drawer of a particular filing cabinet. These filing systems are physical devices that can be simulated by a simple computer program called a *file management system*. Keep in mind, however, that a Rolodex file is a means of retrieving data that are duplicated in the chart. This is an example of the redundancy of data storage that occurs in a physical system.

COMMON STEPS IN USING DATABASE MANAGEMENT SYSTEMS

Imagine a Rolodex deck that is alphabetized by patient last name. One also needs to look up patients by their identification number. One way to do this would be to photocopy every card in the first Rolodex deck, cut out the identification number line, paste it at the top of a new blank card and paste in the remainder underneath. Then one would have to place the new cards in order by sequence of identification numbers and insert them into a second Rolodex holder. This procedure seems a little absurd, but it points out the limitations of a system that depends on a physical layout to organize data. A computerized file management system would do this electronically. It would have all the data in one list, and the user could electronically and quickly create both formats.

File management systems are the simplest of several forms of database management systems. Figure 1 schematically represents the common features of all database management systems: (1) a method of defining the data that will be stored and the data organization; (2) a method of data entry and editing; and (3) a form of retrieval. The first step, data definition and organization, is most important because it establishes what data will be stored and it restricts how the data will be available for analysis later.

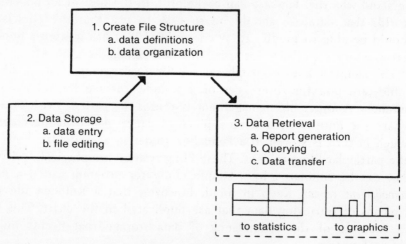

Figure 1. Steps in using database management.

Consider the example of laboratory tests that might be ordered in a psychopharmacology unit. It would be important to list all the different tests (defining what the data will be), and to lay out the format for the data (whether all their numbers would be whole numbers or decimals, and where the decimal points would be placed). Then it would be necessary to define the content of each item (e.g., the range of a lithium level, including upper and lower bounds). Finally, after defining the data items, one needs to take this list of data items and organize it into a database structure. Even in creating a Rolodex file we have to decide what the row and column of each item should be. Defining the file structure in the computer is analagous to this.

The second step in using a database requires some form of data entry. This could utilize the keyboard, an optical scanning device, or a voice recognition unit, but what is important is that one has a way of entering the values and then checking their consistency with the data definition. We want to capture quality data. This is most important in a research database, and the system needs to be able to check for the correctness of data in form and in content, as well as to identify omissions. If data are missing on a patient in a research study, one needs some way of going back and putting it in later. This introduces the third step common to all databases, retrieval.

Retrieval is the means by which a body of stored data is tapped to generate a variety of different reports, organized in different ways without the redundancy of retyping the original data. This is possible because the program can reorganize data with relative independence from any physical layout. The location of any individual piece of data is indicated internally as a symbolic reference point rather than as a physical reference point. This makes it possible to do a very useful function called sorting.

As an example, consider a study in which 35 children were treated with the drug desipramine for over one year. The investigators gathered data from histories, mental status exams, laboratory tests, vital signs, and rating scales. They coded the data numerically and entered it each week as they gathered it, so patient number one had an entry made in week number one and so did patients number two and three. In the second week, patient number one had a second entry, but patient number four had his first entry. This is a simple chronologic sequence of data entry. At the end of the study, the investigators needed to rearrange the order of that information for analysis, so they asked the program to sort the data in a couple of different ways. They asked that all six-year-olds be reported first. In that list of six-year-olds, they asked for all the patients to be listed alphabetically by last name, so the child with the last name of Abel had his whole file listed first. Within each child's set of data, each visit was listed chronologically (first visit listed first, then second and third visit). The program then retrieved the data from the next child, Brown, and when it reported all the six-year-olds, then it retrieved the seven-year-olds. This illustrates how sorting can be done in a variety of ways and levels. A more powerful program offers more sorting functions.

MAJOR TYPES OF DATABASE MANAGEMENT SYSTEMS AND THEIR FEATURES

Having briefly described the three major steps in database management systems, it is worthwhile to examine the limitations of storing data by a somewhat rigid file structure. Often it is necessary or desirable to save different categories of data in different files. Figure 2a shows a database structured into two different tables or files with two different types of data. The first file contains demographic data on each patient and the second contains treatment data from each visit. This represents the nature of different files in a file management type of database management system. If one wanted to track a patient's medication from the visit table and match it with his or her age and sex, a file management type of system would be inadequate. For clinical data, one really needs the freedom to create multiple files while still being able to relate one element in one file to another element in another file, as in figure 2b. To relate data from two different lists one needs a *relational database management system*. Relational systems allow one to change the relationships between data fields after the initial format is laid out and even after much data has been stored in the system.

PATIENT FILE

ID#	NAME	SEX	DOB	MD
001	Jones, Frank	M	02/09/29	Dr. Green
009	Brown, Lynn	F	11/30/54	Dr. Gold
378	Doe, Donald	M	09/18/44	Dr. Dow
....	......, ...	....	.../.../...	....

VISIT FILE

ID#	VISIT	DATE	MEDICATION	DOSE
001	1	01/03/85	lithium carbonate	1200 mg
001	2	01/10/85	lithium carbonate	900 mg
009	9	01/10/85	amitryptyline	150 mg
....	.....	.../.../...	....	....

Figure 2a. Patient and Visit Files.

PATIENT FILE

ID#	NAME	SEX	DOB	MD
001	Jones, Frank	M	02/09/29	Dr. Green
009	Brown, Lynn	F	11/30/54	Dr. Gold
378	Doe, Donald	M	09/18/44	Dr. Dow
....	......, ...	....	.../.../...	....

VISIT FILE

ID#	VISIT	DATE	MEDICATION	DOSE
001	1	01/03/85	lithium carbonate	1200 mg
001	2	01/10/85	lithium carbonate	900 mg
009	9	01/10/85	amitryptyline	150 mg
....	.....	.../.../...	....	....

Figure 2b. Patient and Visit Files.

The flexibility of being able to change these relationships is usually an advantage, but there is one relationship that should never be changed, and that is the relationship of any particular data element to time. Since patients are treated over time and they respond over time, any particular lab test or therapeutic intervention should always be forced to relate to time first and to anything else choosen secondarily. A relational database management system can flexibly relate different items within two lists, but one that fixes these relationships among data elements from the outset is called a *hierarchical database management system*.

A hierarchical database imposes a hierarchy of relationships among data fields. When a hierarchical database is designed to fix the relationship of all items with respect to time, then it is called a *time-oriented database management system*. From the foregoing discussion it becomes clear that a time-oriented database management system is optimal for building a clinical database.

Figure 3 represents three different lists of data items. The arrows indicate that the identification number of the patient in the demographic list is related symbolically to that patient's visits in the visit list, and that those visits are related to laboratory tests in the third list. So, compared to the two-dimensional database of separate files in figure 2a, figure 3 shows a database composed of multiple interconnected files and therefore is three-dimensional.

These are the fundamental differences among the file management system, the hierarchical, relational, and time-oriented database management systems. The easiest programs to learn are file management

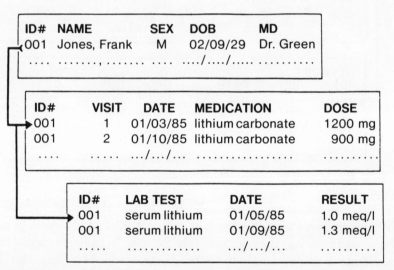

Figure 3. Relational database. The arrows indicate that relations can be drawn among data fields in different files, creating a three-dimensional file structure.

systems, but they are not flexible enough for most needs. Of the relational database management systems, the most celebrated is dBase. dBase has been revised repeatedly, and is flexible and powerful. It is easy to use for simple things, but for more complex things it is almost as difficult to learn as a programming language. Hierarchical systems tend to be easier to use than relational systems.

Integration is an important feature appearing in newer database software. Integration simply means that the program combines database management, graphics, and statistical analysis. Lotus 1–2–3 is the most commercially successful integrated database management system. It is hierarchical but not time-oriented nor particularly powerful. Medlog is another integrated package designed as a medical time-oriented database management system that integrates statistics and to some extent graphics (Layard, 1983). An integrated database management system is particularly useful because once the user generates the tabulated output, he can then directly transfer it into a statistical analysis program without having to retype all the data into a separate program. Without this integrated function, one must either retype data into a separate statistical analysis program manually, or transfer it through an electronic file transfer system.

Finally, any discussion of clinical database systems should include File Manager, developed by the Veterans Administration (Gastfriend et al., 1984). File Manager is not a file management system, despite the similarity in name. File Manager is a sophisticated, hierarchical, time-oriented database management system that offers multiuser capability.

File Manager's multiuser capability is possible because of a function called file lock-out. File lock-out is necessary in the situation where more than one person tries to access a file at the same time. This happens when a secretary wants to update a patient's fee and, at the same time, the physician wants to update something in the clinical progress note. Without file lock-out, the secretary "takes the file out" electronically, opens it up, and updates the balance. Meanwhile, the doctor finishes his note and wants to put it into the place where the file is supposed to be. If the database program lacks the file lock-out procedure, it will dump that doctor's note into an imaginary electronic place and mangle or permanently lose that information. File lock-out prevents this by first updating the fee while "holding" the doctor's note momentarily. Then once the fee is updated, the note is released or unlocked, to be entered into the file. This happens in an instant and the two simultaneous users need not know about it; it is an essential ingredient for a multiuser database management system.

Security is another important function for multiuser clinical databases. With multiple users, there is a need for multiple levels of security. A secretary should have an identification code, or key, that gives access to demographic information, insurance, and fiscal information, but not to all of the clinical information. Clinicians need access to all the clinical information, but if there is a research study ongoing in the unit, clinicians should be kept blind to patients' placebo or drug status. Only the project coordinator should have the security code number that gives that access. Finally, the unit chief alone needs access to administrative data such as the productivity reports for all clinicians.

Another feature of File Manager, unlike most multiuser systems, is that it is a "programmerless" system. In order to create a file structure, File Manager interviews the clinician, in a question and answer dialogue, prompting for each piece of data: What would you like to call that piece of data? How long should it be? Should it be numbers? Should it be letters? Where in the sequence of data would you like to put it? File Manager offers a help response at each step, enabling even nonprogrammers to tell the computer exactly how to electronically create this file. Instead of embroiling the user in the intricacies of a programming language, this programmerless system lets clinicians design their database in plain English.

COMPARING DATABASE NEEDS IN RESEARCH VERSUS CLINICAL CARE

Having described the steps common to all databases, as well as some fundamental features distinguishing different database programs, consider the differences in using a program for research purposes as opposed to clinical ones. A research database management system has an easier job. One reason is that the data are defined prospectively: scales and lab data to be gathered will be selected in advance, and every subject should have the same variables gathered. Data items are usually numeric and they will usually all be the same length. Since a study has only so many subjects and no more, the entire file should be finite in size. At the end of the study one can take all the forms, type them in and perform an analysis all at once, in batch. Finally, a research project will have a limited number of users for its particular database.

A clinical database management system is completely different. First of all, data may change. By the time Mrs. Jones has been seen for four years, her anxiety disorder may have a different diagnosis because *DSM-III-Revised* will have undergone revision. Different variables are gathered for every patient. A patient on tricyclic antidepressants who complains of postural dizziness will get orthostatic blood pressures recorded, while another patient may not. Some of the patient information may be entered in plain English sentences, or free text form. Dictated paragraphs may need to be transcribed into the system or typed in directly by clinicians. Free text fields are always of variable length. Some patients might require half a page, just to describe the history of present illness, while others might require only two sentences. The feature that enables a program to take a data element like a free text field and variably compress or enlarge the electronic space needed to store it is called sparse field handling. Sparse field handling is an essential feature in a clinical database system, because otherwise one would have to specify in advance how big a record would be, how many bytes, kilobytes, or megabytes of storage each patient must have allotted to his file. This would waste so much space in most cases that it would be prohibitively expensive.

A clinical record is constantly growing. After a period of years it needs summarizing to remain useful. Actually, this is one great potential use of the computer. Data entry and output need to be immediate. Immediate availability is also called real time, as opposed to batch processing. Finally, clinical records are used by a multitude of people, from the secretary to the social worker to the psychiatrist, and often two or more users may need a record simultaneously. Two people in two different sites may be using the same chart. Also, users change over time, such as residents who rotate through a program. All of these needs distinguish a clinical database system from a research system, and they demand much more sophisticated features. These differences suggest why implementation of clinical databases has been so formidable, despite the success of computerized research databases. An excellent review on the problems of clinical databases is presented by Hedlund, Vieweg, and Cho (1985) in the premier issue of *Computers and Human Services*.

COMPUTERIZED DATABASES FOR IMPROVED CLINICAL CARE

Despite the complex challenge of implementation, clinical databases have been shown to improve care in a number of ways. It comes as no surprise that secretarial staff can be made more efficient by automating many tasks. Electronic files can reduce redundant tasks while also reducing the rate of human error. Clinical databases (see figure 4) have been able to eliminate transcription by enabling physicians to enter their own evaluations (Hale & Delaune, 1984). Other tangible benefits have been automated reports and scheduling.

The clinical record itself can be made more legible and organized through computerization. Also, the computerized database can be made to provide summary reports of longitudinal patient data, such as treatment response to medication. Unlike the conventional paper record, the computer can present such information more clearly

---

Secretarial Staff Efficiency:
  decrease redundant tasks
  reduce rate of human error
  speed/eliminate transcription
  automate reports & scheduling

Case Management:
  issue patient reminders & recall
  remind MDs of their own protocols
  automate & check workups

Clinical Record:
  increase legibility, organization,
    summarization, graphic
    display
  improve access to records

Quality Assurance & Continuing Education:
  help MDs organize data collection
  track adequacy of data collection
  question exceptional prescribing
  "second opinion" diagnoses

Figure 4. How clinical databases can improve care.

and in a graphic mode as well. Improved access to records, even by multiple simultaneous users, has been described above.

In case management it is often helpful but difficult to call patients who need follow-up (e.g., monthly lithium levels or medication refills). The computer can generate a personalized letter easily at less cost than a secretary. At the Brigham and Women's Hospital in Boston, staff in an outpatient primary care medical unit either telephoned patients to remind them of appointments or sent a computer-generated letter reminder or no reminder at all. They reported that whether they telephoned the patients (human voice) or sent them a reminder letter, the no-show rate dropped from 24% to 14% (Bigby et al., 1983).

A database has also proven useful in reminding physicians of their own treatment protocols. Internists at the Regenstreif Institute in Indiana had their own treatment protocols (tests and procedures to include in routine care) programmed into the computerized medical record. When the doctors deviated from their own protocol, the computer issued them a reminder and they responded to it. The feedback made the system seem useful to them and it became a popular tool (McDonald et al., 1984). A different outcome is described in this volume by Ericson at the Institute of Living, where the lithium treatment protocol issued physicians reminders to have various tests done before lithium could be administered to hospitalized patients. That system was not readily accepted and lasted only two months. Even an effective database function such as physician reminders may not be accepted in all settings.

In quality assurance as well as in continuing education there are a number of studies reporting computerized clinical database systems to be useful. At the University of Vermont, residents were required to enter their clinical workups on every hospitalized patient into a clinical information system that audits their workups for missing clinical history or laboratory data and tells the residents what they missed. The residents showed a striking improvement in the completeness of their workups. This happened most dramatically in the first year of training and it remained consistent throughout three years of residency.

Clinical databases have also been used to question exceptional prescribing. At the Rockland Research Institute, a pharmacy database program issued notes to psychiatrists whenever they were prescribing two similar agents (e.g., Thorazine and Haldol) to the same patient, or when they were using dosages that were either too low or too high relative to established guidelines. Even before the system became operational (just on the basis of announcement letters), the proportion of exceptional prescribing began to diminish. As the computer began to issue letters notifying psychiatrists of their exceptional prescriptions, the number of these exceptions plummeted steadily. This is a convincing test of the computerized database's usefulness in improving patient care by directly changing the behavior of clinicians (Laska, Siegel, & Simpson, 1980).

A final example of the usefulness of databases is second opinion diagnosis. When Greist's group at the University of Wisconsin offered psychiatrists a program to analyze patients' symptoms and signs, the second opinion given by the computer was not well accepted. In another version, also developed by Greist et al. (1983), but tested at The Carrier Foundation, patients were diagnosed by direct computer interview (Mathieson et al., 1985). Although the physicians had already made their own diagnosis, they found the second opinion reached by the computer to be helpful in more than half of the cases because the computer either confirmed their diagnosis or it gave them additional diagnoses that they had not considered.

CONCLUSION

Computerized database management systems have existed for over 25 years, yet they have achieved only minimal acceptance in mental health applications. Several factors can be blamed for this prolonged "gestation" period, including the complexity of the clinical record, the lack of ease in using available software tools, and inflated expectations. The storage of clinical data is much more complex than research database management. Nevertheless, the microcomputer revolution has put newer software tools within reach of psychiatrists and psychologists that are easier to use and yet sophisticated enough for the complex tasks of clinical data storage.

Numerous advantages of computerizing clinical records have been demonstrated, including increased office efficiency, improved organization and access to records, better case management, quality assurance, and medical training. Although effective applications have not been accepted in every installation, the computer has passed several tests of its ability to influence clinicians' behavior for better clinical care. While further development of useful clinical applications of computerized databases continues, the goal for future work will be to combine successful applications into integrated systems that will serve as routine tools for daily use by mental health clinicians.

REFERENCES

Anderson, H. 1984. Letter to the editor. *New England Journal of Medicine* 311(18): 1189.

Barnett, G. O. 1984a. Letter to the editor. *New England Journal of Medicine* 311(18): 1189.

———. 1984b. The application of computer-based medical-record systems in ambulatory practice. *New England Journal of Medicine* 310(25): 1643–1650.

Bigby, J. A., J. Giblin, E. M. Pappius, L. Goldman. 1983. Appointment reminders to reduce no-show rates. *Journal of The American Medical Association* 250(13): 1742–1745.

Friedman, R. B., and D. A. Gustafson. 1977. Computers in clinical medicine, a critical review. *Computers and Biomedical Research* 10:199–203.

Gastfriend, D. R., L. Baer, A. Bhatty, and J. F. Rosenbaum. 1984. Software considerations in the development of an integrated clinical/research database in psychopharmacology. *Computers in Psychiatry/Psychology* 6(2): 19–22.

Greist, J. H., M. H. Klein, H. P. Erdman, and J. W. Jefferson. 1983. Computers and psychiatric diagnosis. *Psychiatric Annals* 13:785–792.

Hale, M. S. and W. DeLaune. 1983. Microcomputer use on a consultation-liaison service. *Psychosomatics* November 24(11): 1003–1015.

Hedlund, J. L., B. W. Vieweg, and D. W. Cho. 1985. Mental health computing in the 1980s: I. General information systems and clinical documentation. *Computers in Human Services* 1(1): 3–33.

Houser, W. A. 1984. End user software engineering: The experience of the Veterans Administration decentralized hospital computer program. *M.U.G. Quarterly* 13(3): 3–11.

Laska, E. M., C. Siegel, and G. M. Simpson. 1980. An automated review system for orders of psychotropic drugs. *Archives of General Psychiatry* 37:824–827.

Layard, M. W. 1983. Medlog: a microcomputer-based clinical data management system. In AAMSI Congress 83, *Proceedings of the Congress on Medical Informatics,* ed. D. A. B. Lindberg, E. E. Van Brunt, and M. A. Jenkins. 464–468.

Mathiesen, K. S., F. J. Evans, K. Meyers, J. M. Rochford, G. F. Wilson, and R. K. Goodstein. 1985. *Interactive computerized DIS (DSM-III) Diagnosis.* Unpublished paper. Carrier Clinic Foundation, Belle Mead, NJ.

McDonald, E. J., S. L. Hui, D. M. Smith, W. M. Tierney, S. J. Cohen, M. Weinberger, and G. P. McCabe. 1984. Reminders to physicians from an introspective computer medical record. *Annals of Internal Medicine* 100:130–138.

Pryor, D. B., R. M. Califf, F. R. Harrell, M. A. Hlatky, K. L. Lee, D. B. Mark, and R. A. Rosati. 1984. *Clinical databases—accomplishments and unrealized potential.* Paper presented at National Center for Health Services Research. Savannah, GA, October 16–19.

Wiederhold, G. 1981. *Databases for Health Care.* New York: Springer-Verlag.

Young, D. W. 1984. What makes doctors use computers?: discussion paper. *Journal of The Royal Society of Medicine* 77:663–667.

PART IV

COMPUTERIZED MANAGEMENT INFORMATION SYSTEMS

9

USE OF COMPUTERS IN MENTAL HEALTH MANAGEMENT OF INFORMATION

James Robinson

What are the uses of a mental health information system? How can you ensure that a mental health information system is useful? There are no standard answers to these questions. The uses of an information system and the methods for ensuring usefulness are idiosyncratic to each organization. Furthermore, these questions can be answered only by the organization asking them.

There is, however, a logical, straightforward, and simple strategy for examining and/or developing a mental health information system that will facilitate positive answers to the questions.

The strategy can be delineated as a series of steps as follows:

Determine objectives

Determine general uses

Specify content or data elements

Determine software characteristics

Select software and hardware

Procurement or development

Careful determination of the objectives (major functions) and proposed uses of a mental health information system will allow the content or specific data required of the system to be extrapolated. It is only then that the questions of software and hardware can be addressed, and of the two, software is the more important consideration. How the software is used—for example, its operational characteristics—is most important. Software systems for use in mental health environments exist for every level of computer: micro, mini, and mainframe. In addition, enough technology exists so that all sorts of configurations can be accommodated: stand-alone micro-, mini-, or mainframe computers; microcomputers attached to mini- or mainframe computers so that data can pass back and forth for larger scale processing; and mini- and/or mainframe computers with many terminals and/or a mix of terminals and microcomputers.

A few key points should be kept in mind when following this process:

1. As many people from your organization as is feasible should be involved in determining the objectives, uses, and content.

2. Definition of the objectives and uses of the system requires a detailed analysis and understanding of the information needs of the entire organization.

3. Use and content decisions should not be made without significant input from potential users of the information system.

4. The objectives and uses of the information system should not focus on current uses but on uses projected for a minimum of three to five years into the future.

5. Human factors—the people aspect of the system—must be considered. What types of people, at what level, and in what jobs will use and operate the system.

In general, the objectives and uses of a system should parallel the information needs of an organization. If information needs match properly planned uses of the system, then the system will be useful, successful and, in all likelihood, cost-effective for the organization.

GENERAL USES OF A MENTAL HEALTH INFORMATION SYSTEM

The number of uses for a system is limited only by imagination. Some of the major uses are:

Record Keeping. Maintain patient, personnel, and fiscal data for day-to-day operations, management decision making, and instant use in emergency room care.

Reporting. Produce reports for federal, state, and local government agencies, for accrediting agencies, and for internal needs.

Billing. Account for services received, maintain fee schedules by type of service, produce bills.

Quality Assurance. Develop and monitor care standards/norms, monitor program change, produce case review data.

Program Evaluation. Monitor service utilization, process and outcome, analyze trends and program change.

Personnel. Schedule appointments, keep track of shift, work locations and staff assignments.

Productivity. Analyze personnel utilization and costs, review staff assignments and service delivery patterns.

Planning. Utilize data on current operations to plan in programmatic and fiscal arenas.

Research. Study questions of importance to your agency using a standard data set.

GENERAL CONTENT AREAS OF A MENTAL HEALTH INFORMATION SYSTEM

Mental health information system software packages are available from many vendors. The content of each is different so that a buyer must have an understanding of objectives and proposed uses in the agency in order to choose the system that will be most useful. If an organization is planning to develop a mental health information system (which is not usually recommended), then the precise objectives, uses, and content of the system must be known for systems development to proceed expeditiously and cost-effectively. One of the most frequent mistakes made by buyers/developers of mental health information systems is the failure to give enough cognizance (at least when considering an automated information system) to the fact that the real business of mental health organizations is providing patient care. Just as the core activity of a mental health organization is patient care, patient information is the core component of any mental health information system. Administrative, business, fiscal, and revenue systems are critical components of a mental health information system, but these components should be constructed around the patient information system core.

The uses of a mental health information system are far too comprehensive to discuss adequately within the scope of this paper. Presented below is a brief overview of the general uses and content areas of a mental health information system that should be considered. It should be noted that each general area might contain dozens of individual pieces of data.

PATIENT

Patient Tracking

In a mobile society where patients may appear for service at many locations within a delivery network, the ability to track patients to ensure continuity and quality of care becomes a primary goal. A computer system can allow authorized personnel immediate access to record data no matter where or when the patient has been seen previously. Of course, tracking also depends upon unique identifiers for each patient, which can come in the form of identification numbers, codes dependent on the spelling of names and other data. Thus, once a patient's name, number, or some other identifying mechanism is entered, the computer should, in fact, be able to tell you whether or not that particular patient has ever received treatment from your organization and/or perhaps from other organizations with which you have collaborative data sharing agreements with suitable confidentiality and privacy protection. Even more important, if that particular patient or client has been in the system, historical data should immediately be available to you (assuming that you are permitted legally to have access to those data).

Case Registry

If information about patients is being processed, then a case registry should automatically be available. The case registry should list the name of the patient and some other pertinent facts, such as identification number or date of birth. A good case registry is, in fact, a guide to finding a case record when little is known about the patient. By providing rapid access to the records, the case registry reduces data entry activities, since only new data need be added, and allows rapid review of the case history to determine treatment strategies.

Admission/Registration Demographics

A wide range of data can be collected and stored on the computer. The admission/registration process should create the computerized record, store the data, and update the case registry. Identifying and demographic data required by the organization should be collected during the admission/registration process.

Location/Movement

Physical location data keep track of patients as they move through a facility and/or through a service delivery network. A system should be able to track patients in physical locations as well as in many programs simultaneously.

Responsible Persons

A system should record the case manager and/or the clinicians assigned to various aspects of care.

Appointment Scheduling

An appointment scheduling system allows you to schedule patient appointments for clinicians and patients, recording which patients are coming, for what service, at what time, and for how long. If you do appointment scheduling and add to it a mechanism verifying that the appointment was kept as planned or changed, you can significantly reduce the work required for services recording, one of the most labor-intensive aspects of a mental health information system. Since most of the data is already in the computer, only the changes need be added.

Services

Complete and accurate documentation of service delivery, including consultation, education, and administrative activities, is essential to many administrative, case management, and reporting functions. Using an appointment scheduling system to facilitate service recording is one way of proceeding; however, agencies that keep their appointment schedules manually may enter into the computer all the data concerning services and activities. Usually, manually kept activity logs are the sources of the data. Services recording contains the exact information needed for regulatory reporting, billing, budgeting and planning.

Placement/Referral

Information on placement or referral is needed for aftercare, for outcome studies and for follow-up.

Drugs

Drug systems allow you to enter every drug order prescribed for a patient. A formulary component acts to ensure that the drugs prescribed are, in fact, those that are available within the organization. Pharmacy operations and inventory control should also be part of a drug system.

Treatment Planning

The system should facilitate the recording and monitoring of the treatment planning cycle: evaluating the case, setting treatment goals, prescribing treatment strategies, evaluating their success.

Assessments

Evaluating a patient at admission to get baseline data and subsequently to determine progress and to review treatment strategies is essential. Assessments on many dimensions should be available, such as level of care, mental status, and diagnosis.

Quality Assurance/Clinical Policy Monitoring

Accreditation, regulatory, and funding agencies require services delivery organizations to adhere to accepted standards of practice.

Monitoring the delivery process becomes an administrative responsibility in which some areas are amenable to computer assistance. For example, a quality assurance system associated with a drug system can monitor prescribing policies, with regard to dose ranges, polypharmacy issues, allergies, and previous adverse reactions. One of the things the computer does very well is to remember things. Once you put in a data item, such as a patient's allergy to a specific medication, or a specific combination of medications to be avoided, the computer can be asked to inform you when such an event might occur or has occurred. Notice that the computer is not making a decision. The computer is merely comparing the incoming data with policies or quality-of-care issues that the organization wants noted. In this way, the computer helps review committees oversee that quality-of-care policies set by your organization are adhered to. With medications, this process happens to be relatively easy. Extending monitoring to less-well-defined areas is much more difficult. Development of monitoring rules/guidelines/criteria has yet to be done. Although the software developed for medication monitoring is generalizable, more work is needed in other clinical areas.

Billing/Accounting

Billing and accounting systems should prepare bills for all types of payers including federal, private, third party, self-pay, and other claims. The system should create an account for each patient, prepare bills, post revenues, and audit accounts. It should also facilitate DRG financial reporting, bad-debt management, revenue analysis, payment analysis by payer, and posting to a general ledger system.

Discharge

A discharge system should allow the recording of the facts surrounding termination of service: reason for discharge, referral, if any, to what agency, the type of agency, address, the contact person and telephone number, and follow-up to find out if the patient got there.

Agency Defined/Idiosyncratic Data

The system should be able to accomodate the special data needs of your own setting without extensive programming changes.

BUSINESS/FISCAL

General Ledger

The general ledger is the core component of the automated business/fiscal system. It enables organizations to establish and maintain a chart of accounts, post all standard bookkeeping entries, produce financial statements, and close the books at the end of the fiscal period. The general ledger also serves as the hub around which the other components or modules of the business/fiscal system (e.g. payroll, accounts payable) are added.

Payroll

The main functions of the payroll module are to produce payroll checks and to provide reports that summarize internal cost allocations (i.e., personnel costs by location) and reports that summarize state and federal tax liabilities for the period and for the fiscal year.

Human Resources Management

Whereas the function of the payroll module is to produce payroll checks and to provide information summarizing state and federal tax liabilities, the human resource management system is designed to provide supplemental employee information useful to managers at both the program and agency levels.

Accounts Payable

Accounts payable provides an automated system to assist in the control of purchases and payments. The module records purchase transactions, invoices presented for payment, open items and payments made.

OPERATIONAL CHARACTERISTICS

Several characteristics are absolutely imperative to the successful operation of an information system in a mental health organization.

Easy to Use

A system should be usable by staff not necessarily trained in data processing. It should have clear, understandable data entry screens, on-screen prompting and/or assistance, and simple procedures. Data retrieval and inquiry functions should be easy to learn. Documentation and instructional materials should be well written and directed at appropriate staff levels.

Comprehensive and Integrated

The goal is to have patient, fiscal, and administrative data within one system. The crucial element here is a database management system that stores the information and makes it available for use when needed. Many available packages can produce screens and accept data; however, these data may be useless unless they are managed and stored in such a way as to be available to retrieval packages, inquiry functions, and other processing needs. For example, information on services delivered to a patient is needed by the billing programs and must be stored so as to facilitate that access.

Flexible and Dynamic

You should have the ability to change any system you are considering and to adapt it to meet your organizational and data processing requirements, not vice versa. That means you should be able to add things into existing content areas; you should be able to add new content areas; and you should be able to put in your own applications with minimal data processing expertise.

Interactive

The system should allow direct key data entry, immediate editing, processing, and permanent storage. In addition, access to that system should be in the hands of the people generating the data. Data entry devices, whether microcomputers or other terminals, should be placed where the data are going to be collected, so correction can be made at the original source of the data. Terminals will not just be used for data entry; they will also be used to retrieve information, to look at information so that the mental health management information system becomes an integral part of the day-to-day operation of the organization.

Menu Driven

Most systems today are menu driven. What that means is that you get a set of choices on the screen: admit a patient; look at some data (inquiry); schedule appointments; or generate reports. You then select what you want to do. Menu driven systems allow the use of the system to be directly under the control of the users.

Retrieval

Getting the data in is easy; the problem is often getting information out. There are several different types of information retrieval.

Inquiry

Most systems allow inquiry, with the results appearing on video display screens. You want to be able to go in and look at anything entered into the system, at any detail you want, over any historical period. Both current and historical information stored in computer files should be displayed instantly on the video display terminal for viewing by authorized personnel. On most computers today, anything that you see on the screen can automatically be printed with the push of one or two buttons.

Standard Reports

There should be menus and standard reports available in any mental health information system. These should be easy to generate and require little if any data processing expertise.

Do-It-Yourself Reports

The mental health environment is replete with regulatory requirements from numerous agencies. Service providers must meet these reporting requirements, which change frequently. You cannot be dependent on a vendor to help you meet new requirements. Within your system, you must have some tools that allow you to design and create your own reports. There really are only three general types of reports: listings, tables, and statistical analyses. Generalized retrieval packages should be capable of producing all three types of reports and should be usable by personnel with little or no data processing expertise. Microcomputers have much more limited generalized retrieval packages. In many cases, micros do not have the power to do the large mathematical and statistical routines.

The capability of creating diskettes and/or tapes for intermediary billing agencies or to meet regulatory reporting requirements is important.

Access Control

Make sure any system you consider has rigid security to protect the confidentiality of the data and privacy of the patients.

Growth

Mental health organizations need a system that will grow with the organization; do not pick or develop a system that merely meets your needs today. When selecting a system, look at future needs; you do not want to be changing systems every year or two. In many cases it is more difficult to move from one automated system to another than from a manual to an automated system.

Support Services

Vendors must be available to service both software and hardware products when they do not function properly, to answer questions about their products, and to provide training in the use of their products. Costs of support services must be included in budgeting for an information system, as maintenance and service contracts are a necessity.

CHOOSING HARDWARE

The hardware trails your decision on software. Do not go out and buy a computer and then say, I'd like a mental health management information system; let's see what software runs on this particular computer. That is the wrong way to do it. Decide what your system should be, then look for software packages that meet these needs. When you have done that, you can then choose the computer to run the software. Done in reverse, the agency may end up with a computer that is not suited to the desired system.

Although there are no guarantees that a mental health information system will be useful and successful, systematic and careful planning will increase

> the likelihood that the system will meet objectives and expected information needs

> the probability of successful use of the system and

> the probability that your system will be a cost-effective investment.

Ensuring that a mental health information system is useful is no different than ensuring that a house is useful. First, you must have the right foundation: setting objectives, determining uses in advance and selecting content. The structure is the software, which rests upon the foundation. Hardware is required to complete the structure.

If properly constructed on a solid foundation, given proper ongoing attention and maintenance, your mental health information system will last for years, and its use will be limited only by imagination and fiscal resources.

10

CLINICAL APPLICATIONS OF COMPUTERIZED MANAGEMENT INFORMATION SYSTEMS

Peter Ericson

Not too many years ago when I spoke about computers at conferences, there were few who attended and they were interested in *what* could be done with the computer. This has changed. Now what people want to know is *how* can *they* use the computer. Most of you understand very well what can be done with the computer because you have microcomputers yourselves. Here I will discuss what we are doing at the Institute of Living. This will provide insight into what can be done, based on our experience over quite a few years.

To put my observations in perspective, I will identify the resources that we have at the Institute of Living (you will see we are not a microcomputer installation), describe the direction that we are heading in, and discuss our comprehensive clinical database, providing examples of how we use it with our Clinical Information Abstract and the Lithium Protocol System. I will also refer to some of the problems that we have experienced and some of the solutions.

The Institute of Living has a long history, as does our use of computers. We started, thanks to the foresight of Dr. Bernard Glueck, who was the director of research, in the early sixties. He was able to obtain a National Institute of Mental Health grant that lasted for five years, specifically to see how computers might be used to aid clinicians in psychiatry. We developed a Hospital Information System in 1967. We now have a Tandem computer. This is a nonstop system often used by banks, because there is no single point of failure in the computer system. We will shortly have four CPUs with 10 megabytes of memory and 12 disk drives with a total of three gigabytes of on-line storage. We have access to only half of that because we use mirroring, where all data are recorded redundantly. We have 67 CRTs, 20 printing terminals, and six microcomputers, all networked. We have a coaxial network. We use four different languages; COBOL, FORTRAN, BASIC, and MUMPS, as well as a programmerless system called Fileman, which will be discussed later in the chapter. There is a staff of 20, the system cost about a million dollars, and our annual budget is $850,000. Again, to put things in perspective, we are not working with a microcomputer.

In 1967 our hospital information system had one CPU, the IBM 1440. Its maximum memory was 16k. It had three disk drives with a total of six megabytes. We had eight CRTs and one language, Autocoder. Some of the good things that we were doing with that system we are not doing today. This reflects on the capability of the people as opposed to the hardware. While there are some things you cannot do unless you have certain hardware, I know we could still be productive with the 1967 system as far as developing useful applications is concerned.

We all know that information is power and that it is important for us to recognize it as a resource. In our hospital, the primary mission is patient care, provided by the clinical staff. Secondary missions are research and education. The resources that support these missions fall into four categories; fiscal, plant and equipment, human, and information.

We use the acronym IMIS, which stands for Integrated Medical Information Service. This helps us as we try to provide for the future. We have broken down the activity areas into another acronym, CARE. It stands for Clinical, Administrative, Research, and Education. We have people on the staff who are specialists in each of these areas and who work with their respective users.

Another concept to recognize is information modalities: text, voice, graph, image, and data. By recognizing them, you have a chance to plan for the future integration of these modalities. The most obvious example of integration would be text and data. If you are going to dictate a progress note using a phone, that information would, through word processing, go into the database. The same database already has items such as chemistry results and pharmacy orders. The computer can then provide the integration, merging the data to provide a progress note that is accurate. At the same time, it simplifies the task to the provider of the progress note. That is one example of integrating information modalities. There is going to be much more of this as the technology becomes available.

We should also recognize the various process types, that is, what can we do with information. You can record, transmit, retain, transform, and retrieve. For our purpose, it is useful to keep this in mind as you try to plan for the total system.

The institute provides services for inpatients, outpatients, day patients, the children's clinic, and the geriatric clinic. The institute is changing dramatically, because we are now providing short-term care. About five years ago, our median length of stay was 150 days. Three years ago we had a median length of stay of 58 days, and it has remained close to this level since then. Because we have been developing computer systems since 1964, we have a comprehensive system that supports all areas from a central site. Figure 1 shows a computer terminal that provides user access to the system. That was a few years ago, but there is no question but that this has to be a microcomputer. In fact, what the central circle is going to be is another microcomputer that is managing the archival database, performing just this specific function.

My main interest has always been in the use of computers in the clinical area. I call business applications necessary evils. However, that evil is becoming more and more necessary, because there are people who want to see the financial data integrated with the patient data. We have a fairly complete financial system. Interestingly

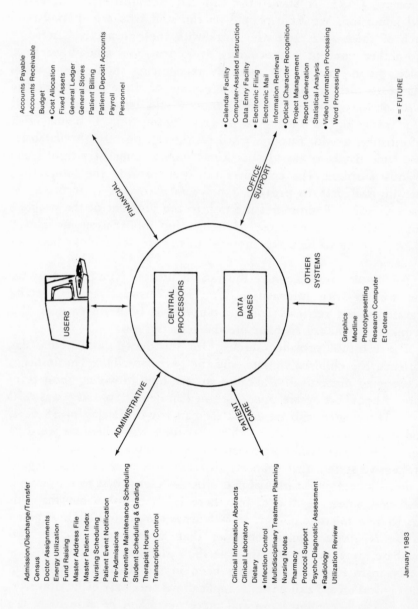

Accounts Payable
Accounts Receivable
Budget
• Cost Allocation
Fixed Assets
General Ledger
General Stores
Patient Billing
Patient Deposit Accounts
Payroll
Personnel

• Calendar Facility
Computer-Assisted Instruction
Data Entry Facility
• Electronic Filing
Electronic Mail
Information Retrieval
• Optical Character Recognition
Project Management
Report Generation
Statistical Analysis
• Video Information Processing
Word Processing

• = FUTURE

FINANCIAL

OFFICE
SUPPORT

USERS

CENTRAL
PROCESSORS

DATA
BASES

OTHER
SYSTEMS

ADMINISTRATIVE

PATIENT
CARE

Graphics
Medline
Phototypesetting
Research Computer
Et Cetera

Admission/Discharge/Transfer
Census
Doctor Assignments
Energy Utilization
Fund Raising
Master Address File
Master Patient Index
Nursing Scheduling
Patient Event Notification
Pre-Admissions
Preventive Maintenance Scheduling
Student Scheduling & Grading
Therapist Hours
Transcription Control

Clinical Information Abstracts
Clinical Laboratory
Dietary
• Infection Control
Multidisciplinary Treatment Planning
Nursing Notes
Pharmacy
Protocol Support
• Psycho-Diagnostic Assessment
• Radiology
Utilization Review

January 1983

Figure I. Institute of Living integrated medical information service inpatient—outpatient—day patient—child.

enough, the one thing that we do not have is cost allocation, but this will be added.

For several years the Veterans Administration has been automating every psychological test that they could find, using MUMPS. I have used their package of tests for several years. At our hospital, however, the staff uses only one out of the whole battery. This is one of the areas that should probably be automated.

Office support is an area of increasing significance because of the cost savings that can be realized. Word processing provides efficiencies. Electronic mail, the ability to transfer information without creating paper, also provides the ability to know who reads the mail, and even addresses the security issue. Our computer produces an enormous amount of paper because we are generating so much information. Much of that information is confidential. Every time it is placed on paper, we are running an unnecessary risk, because if it is in a computer and available only at a terminal, computer security can be utilized.

Our computer is also connected to other systems such as graphics, Medline, phototypesetting, and the research computer for statistical processing. The significance of the clinical database and some of its basic principles must be recognized in order to make data both accurate and timely. We have terminals throughout the hospital, but only one on a unit. A concept that I want to emphasize is the following: The person who knows the information should be the same person who enters the data. Thus a product is produced that they are responsible for. The example that I use is dietary.

Our dietician does a nursing dietary care plan for each patient. After she has interviewed the patient, she provides the information to the computer. The computer then generates a nutritional care plan that comes out on hard copy; she signs it, and it goes into the patient's record. She is responsible for that information. It is in the patient's record, and she produced it. As a result, the database is accurate and timely. That is the key, because one of the things that you cannot do with a stand-alone micro is provide integration of the data. This is extremely important to recognize.

There is so much that you can do with that stand-alone micro that you could keep busy for the next five years, but that is not the issue. You never run out of useful things for the computer to do. What does not always exist is the capability to use the computer to its capacity. One of the requirements for some of our applications is an integrated database with access to information provided from many areas.

Our Clinical Information Abstract (CIA) is one way to "dump" our database (figure 2). It shows the kind of data we routinely collect in our system and how we make it available. It shows administrative data, patient's strengths, problems, current diagnosis and treatment. The sample is not a real patient. The intent is to show all the information that might print for any given patient. The categories include: psychiatric treatment modalities, diagnostic services, physical description, therapeutic visits, objectives and observations, information alerts, statistical indicators, and estimated treatment time available. Most of the content is information that has been collected and is now being printed without change. The report simply provides it in a convenient, timely format. The computer is not doing anything other than retrieving and printing. The last two sections are examples of how the computer can provide added value.

We have 10 different sets of rules that can cause an information alert to print (figure 3, see p. 137). The idea is that whenever we produce one of these Clinical Information Abstracts, which happens at least weekly, the computer is using the criteria to see if this patient's database contains a match. If so, the information alert prints in its section on the CIA. Here we have an example of the computer using information that has been provided and highlighting it in some way, reporting by exception.

The second section is the statistical indicators. In this case, the computer is really reporting information that was not provided. It is creating information. Based on statistics, the system is able to say that this particular patient resembles a group of patients that have done well with a specific treatment. The computer is providing information that might not have been recognized. There may be patients who would not have been considered for a particular treatment.

Another issue is the information versus paper problem. Our clinical lab summary is a good way to make the point. Every time there is a new result, we produce a clinical lab summary sheet (figure 4). There can be three or four pages of lab results for a given patient. If all you want to do is look at the last lithium level, you have four pages of paper when you want to read only one line. That's a problem! On the other hand, there are some people who really want to have access to all of the results when they take a

---

THE INSTITUTE OF LIVING   HARTFORD, CONN.

CLINICAL INFORMATION ABSTRACT   PART I - PAGE 1

38400   MISS JONES, SALLY ·   AGE 21   THERAPIST: MILLER MD, R.   SEC. D

    I. ADMINISTRATIVE

ADMISSION: DATE - 9/22/80 TYPE - FIRST
READMITTED: DATE - 3/12/81 TYPE - DPR
CURRENT UNIT - TODD 1   A LOCKED, INTERMEDIATE UNIT FOR WOMEN 11/28/81
CURRENT ROOM - #12   MULTIPLE OCCUPANCY
> GROUP .... : 9A (11/28/81)
> OBSERVATION...: ROUTINE (11/28/81)
  LEGAL STATUS...: VOLUNTARY   (3/15/81)
  INSURANCE .... : MEDICARE   (A,B)
> MAIL .... : RESTRICTED   (12/01/81)
  STUDENT .... : YES

  UNIT MOVES (PAST 30 DAYS)
>   11/18/81   T THOMPSON 1   A LOCKED, HIGHLY STRUCTURED UNIT FOR WOMEN
>   11/28/81   TODD 1   A LOCKED, INTERMEDIATE UNIT FOR WOMEN

  VISITORS (PAST 30 DAYS)
>   11/20/81   FATHER, MOTHER, SISTER
>   11/27/81   BROTHER
>   11/29/81   MOTHER, SISTER

    II. STRENGTHS

        1. LIKEABLE
        2. APPEARS TO HAVE AT LEAST AVERAGE INTELLIGENCE
        3. FAMILY IS WILLING TO BE INVOLVED IN TREATMENT PLANNING.

    III. PROBLEMS/AREAS OF IMPAIRED FUNCTION
         CURRENT

        1. SLEEP DISTURBANCE
        2. DEPRESSION
        3. LOSS OF AVOCATIONAL INTERESTS

    IV. CURRENT DIAGNOSIS (REVIEW - 10/15/81)

AXIS   CODE   DIAGNOSIS
  I   309.00   ADJUSTMENT DISORDER WITH DEPRESSED MOOD
  II   301.84   (PRIMARY DIAGNOSIS) PASSIVE - AGGRESSIVE PERSONALITY DISORDER
  III   240   - DIABETES MELLITUS
                                                                  (continued)

Figure 2. The Institute of Living, Hartford, Conn. Clinical information abstract.

38400   MISS JONES, SALLY   AGE 21   THERAPIST: MILLER MD, R.   SEC.D

V. TREATMENT
   A. MEDICATION

      1. CURRENT PROFILE

		STANDING ORDERS DUE 12/16/81	ORIGINAL ORDER
WARNING	— NO PILOCARPINE		10/27/81
	— ACETAMINOPHEN 325MGM		09/23/81 QID
	650MGM QID PRN		
CONTROL	— AMYTAL SODIUM 250MGM		9/22/80
	250MGM IM IF PT REFUSES PO		
CONTROL	— AMYTAL 200MGM		8/28/81
	200MGM Q4H PRN SEVERE AGITATION		
	— DIPHENYLHYDANTOIN 100MGM		11/13/81 TID
	100MGM TID		
	— FLAGYL		9/22/80
	1MGM BID		
	— THIORIDAZINE CONCENTRATE 100MGM		9/22/80 QID
	200MGM QID		
	— TRIFLUOPERAZINE CONCENTRATE		8/21/81
	10MGM/ML		
	20MGM BID		
	— ZARONTIN 250MGM		10/15/81 QID
	250 MGM QID		

      2. CANCELLED (PAST 30 DAYS)   CANCELLED

         — ANTACID SUSPENSION   11/28/81 QID
           30ML QID PRN
         — NARDIL 100MGM   11/06/81
           TAKE ONCE A DAY
         — PARNATE 250MGM   11/16/81
           250MGM HS

   B. PSYCHOTHERAPY

      1. GROUP THERAPY

YOUNG ADULT: SRADER, DR. S.   WED 3:00 - 4:30
STARTED: 1/06/82;.: ATTENDED 1, MISSED 0; TOTAL: ATTENDED 8, MISSED 1

   C. SOCIAL SERVICE

SOCIAL WORKER: MONTGOMERY J. (INPATIENTS AND/OR FAMILIES)

   D. DRS WORKSHOPS

TITLE	START	END	REASON
ACTIVITIES OF DAILY LIVING	11/06/81		
DIET AWARENESS	11/21/81	11/25/81	CLASS WAS CANCELLED
SELF-AWARENESS I	10/06/81		
LIFE SKILLS	10/01/81		
EXPRESSIVE MOVEMENT	9/27/81		

38400 MISS JONES, SALLY AGE 21 THERAPIST: MILLER, MD, R. SEC. D

E. DIET

DIET ORDERED: NORMAL 1800-2200 CAL.
DIET-DRUG INTERACTION: NONE   FOOD ALLERGIES: AMERICAN CHEESE
LAST DIETICIAN VISIT: 10/16/81
WEIGHT: 09/80 (ADM) 105   10/81   122   11/81   123   IDEAL: 118

F. SOMATIC THERAPY

CURRENT STATUS	AUTHORIZATION DATES				TREATMENT DATES		TREATMENTS		
	PATIENT	R.P.	COURT	EXEC.	FIRST	LAST	LIM	TOT	WK
COMPLETE	8/14/81	8/13/81	DNA		8/17/81	11/14/81	12	12	0
TOTALS:	BILATERAL 8	UNILATERAL 4							

CHANGE: IDEATION - NO CHANGE   AFFECT - IMPROVED   BEHAVIOR - WORSE
MEMORY LOSS: CONTINUING   SIDE EFFECT: NONE

G. PHYSICAL THERAPY

MODALITY	AFFECTED AREA	DATE	FREQ.	GOAL/STATUS/RESULT
WHIRLPOOL BATH	LEFT WRIST	8/27/81	3/W	PROMOTE HEALING
(CHANGE)		9/03/81	W	
(STATUS)		9/11/81		SLIGHT IMPROVEMENT

VI. ACTIVE PSYCHIATRIC TREATMENT MODALITIES

UNIT PLACEMENT
SPECIAL PRECAUTIONS
MEDICATIONS
PSYCHOTHERAPY   FREQUENCY: 45 MINUTES
DURATION: THREE TIMES PER WEEK

VII. DIAGNOSTIC SERVICES

A. CLINICAL LABORATORY

———————————————— CHEMISTRY ————————————————

	BUN	UR-ACID	PHOS	CA
	8-25	2.3-6.0	0.8-1.5	2.20-2.58
	MG/DL	MG/DL	MMOL/L	MMOL/L
	S=1	S=0.2	S=0.07	S=0.04
> 11/15/81				2.42
> 11/20/81	18	3.87	*1.6	*2.61

ROF = RESULT ON FILE IN MED. REC.   # = MORE RESULTS ON FILE (LAST 5 PRINTED)
  * = RESULTS ABNORMAL AND/OR SIGNIFICANT AND/OR NOT WITHIN THERAPEUTIC RANGE
NOTE: 2 ABNORMAL OCCURRENCES INCLUDED IN NEW RESULTS

(continued)

133

38400   MISS JONES, SALLY   AGE 21   THERAPIST: MILLER MD, R.   SEC. D

B. PSYCHOLOGICAL SERVICES

   1. PSYCHOLOGICAL TESTING

   IQ RESULTS: WECHSLER AT AGE 17

   2. MMPI RESULTS

TYPE	DATE	PROFILE CODE
ADMISSION	9/22/80	8'''972''46'31X
INTERIM	11/24/81	8267'''49''31'X

   3. FIRO-B

DATE	TYPE		INCLUSION	CONTROL	AFFECTION
9/27/80	ADMISSION	EXPRESSED:	1	2	3
		WANTED:	4	5	6
11/06/81	INTERIM	EXPRESSED:	6	5	4
		WANTED:	3	2	1

C. CONSULTATION (PAST 30 DAYS)

   11/12/81 DR. SMITH, SAW PT. ON UNIT
   11/16/81 JEFFERSON X-RAY GROUP
   11/20/81 DR. SMITH SAW PT. ON TH. 1
   11/29/81 DR. FRANKLIN

VIII. SPECIAL BEHAVIOR ACTIVITY (PAST 30 DAYS)

A. REFUSED MEDICATIONS

   11/14/81 DAY SHIFT, 11/16/81 DAY AND NIGHT SHIFTS,
   12/01/81 NIGHT SHIFT, 12/02/81 DAY SHIFT

B. PROTECTIVE RESTRAINTS   (PAST 30 DAYS)

TYPE	DATE	START	STOP	REASON
WET PACK	11/26/81	2:00 AM	5:30 AM	EXTREMELY AGITATED AND ASSAULTIVE

C. SBR: 11/16/81 DAY SHIFT, 11/19/81 NIGHT SHIFT,
           11/24/81 NIGHT SHIFT, 12/02/81 NIGHT SHIFT

IX. PHYSICAL

A. FEMALE   AGE 21   HEIGHT 5'3"   WEIGHT 09/80 (ADM)   105   10/81   122   11/81   123

X. THERAPEUTIC VISITS (PAST 30 DAYS)

   VISIT: 11/22/81   RETURNED: 11/23/81
   VISIT: 11/28/81   RETURNED: 11/30/81

> STATUS CHANGED SINCE LAST PROGRESS NOTE ON 11/05/81

38400   MISS JONES, SALLY   AGE 21   THERAPIST: MILLER MD, R.   SEC. D

I.   CURRENT OBJECTIVES AND OBSERVATIONS

    A. NURSING (11/29/81)

1. BY 2/19, PATIENT WILL BEGIN TO SOCIALIZE WITH THE OTHER PATIENTS ON THE UNIT.
2. BY 3/1, PATIENT WILL BE ABLE TO SLEEP WITHOUT MEDICATION.

    B. REHABILITATIVE SERVICES

        1. TREATMENT PLAN AND GOALS

ENCOURAGE MISS JONES TO ASSUME RESPONSIBILITY FOR HER HOSPITALIZATION, AND TO PLAN AND ORGANIZE ACTIVITIES AS MUCH AS POSSIBLE, ENCOURAGE FOLLOW THROUGH.
    PROVIDE PHYSICAL ACTIVITIES AS A CONSTRUCTIVE OUTLET FOR ENERGY AND STRESS AND TO IMPROVE BODY IMAGE.
    ENCOURAGE EXPRESSION OF THOUGHTS AND FEELINGS AND PROVIDE REALITY ORIENTATION AND CONSTRUCTIVE FEEDBACK TO GAIN INSIGHT.

        2. CURRENT OBJECTIVE (11/19/81)

BY 2/20 PATIENT WILL ATTEND 3 ACTIVITIES PER WEEK. PATIENT WILL ALSO INVOLVE HERSELF IN GROUP ACTIVITIES.

    C. DIETARY

DIET ORDERED: NORMAL 1800-2200 CAL.
DIET-DRUG INTERACTION: NONE   FOOD ALLERGIES: AMERICAN CHEESE
LAST DIETICIAN VISIT: 10/16/81
NUTRITIONAL CONDITION: GOOD
PHYSICAL PROBLEMS: DIABETES MELLITUS
DIET PLAN AND OBJECTIVES:
    TO PREVENT AND ELIMINATE EDEMA THROUGH PROPER DIET.
VISIT PROGRESS NOTES:
    PATIENT STATED THAT SHE ATTENDS THREE MEALS AND HAS A GOOD APPETITE.
LONG TERM GOAL: TO MAINTAIN WEIGHT THROUGH PROPER NUTRITION.
WEIGHT: 09/80 (ADM) 105   10/81   122   11/81   123   IDEAL: 118

REVIEWED BY: _____
           THERAPIST SIGNATURE

38400   MISS JONES, SALLY   AGE 21   THERAPIST: MILLER MD, R.   SEC. D

    I. INFORMATION ALERT

        A. HOSPITAL STANDARD

THIS PATIENT HAS BEEN ON CONTINUOUS (NO D.C. > 2 WEEKS) ANTIPSYCHOTIC MEDICATION FOR LONGER THAN 1 YEAR.

A SEDATIVE MEDICATION HAS BEEN IN EFFECT FOR THIS PATIENT FOR A PERIOD > 2 WEEKS.

(continued)

THIS PATIENT HAS BEEN ON CONTINUOUS (NO D.C. > 2 WEEKS)
ANTIPARKINSON MEDICATION FOR LONGER THAN 3 MONTHS AND
HAS BEEN ON ANTIPSYCHOTIC DRUGS FOR MORE THAN 1 YEAR.

    B. STATISTICAL INDICATORS

THIS PATIENT IS SIMILAR TO A GROUP OF PATIENTS WHO HAVE
RESPONDED WELL TO LITHIUM. MOTION SICKNESS CLASSIFICATION
AND MMPI DATA WERE USED TO FORM THE GROUP.

II. ESTIMATED TREATMENT TIME AVAILABLE FROM DATE OF ADMISSION

    PATIENT INSURED 120 DAYS AT 100%, THEREAFTER.
    DOUBT FAMILY'S ABILITY TO FINANCE 20%.

REPORT NO. 22-6NBU-1 DISTRIBUTION: REQUESTOR

---

look at a new test. This is the continuum that we are all part of. Some people want the minimum, some people want the maximum—how do you know who should have what and when?

Using a paper system, the best that we could come up with is the following: At the bottom, last line of the last page, you can see if there are any abnormals. If abnormal occurrences are reported, another technique is used. All new information on the report is identified by an arrow in the left margin. If all you need to know or all you have time to look at is those abnormals, you look at the bottom line. It shows two abnormals; you scan down for the arrows, and there you find the tests to review. However, one of the biggest complaints from the staff is that there is too much paper in the clinical lab summary. The solution is to get rid of the paper and have a terminal on each clinician's desk. There should be a profile associated with each clinician that would identify how the data should be displayed. With the ability we have now, we can personalize each report. Each person can see just the information he or she wants, which solves the continuum problem.

I was a member of our special studies committee when we did a retrospective study on the use of lithium in the hospital to identify if the proper tests were being done at the right time. I told the committee that with our database we should never have to do that kind of study again. We designed the Protocol Support System. The first use for it was lithium. The way it was designed, the clinician requests a lithium workup sheet that prints all the

1. 12/15/79:	THIS PATIENT HAS BEEN ON CONTINUOUS (NO D.C. > 2 WEEKS) ANTIPSYCHOTIC MEDICATION FOR LONGER THAN 1 YEAR.	6. 3/03/80:	THIS PATIENT HAS A DIAGNOSIS OF MANIC-DEPRESSIVE ILLNESS, MANIC AND HAS BEEN HOSPITALIZED FOR MORE THAN 90 DAYS
2. 3/03/80:	A MINOR TRANQUILIZING AGENT HAS BEEN IN EFFECT FOR THIS PATIENT FOR A PERIOD > 2 WEEKS.	7. 12/15/79:	THIS PATIENT HAS BEEN ON CONTINUOUS (NO D.C. > 2 WEEKS) ANTIPARKINSON MEDICATION FOR LONGER THAN 3 MONTHS AND HAS BEEN ON ANTIPSYCHOTIC DRUGS FOR MORE THAN 1 YEAR.
3. 3/03/80:	A SEDATIVE MEDICATION HAS BEEN IN EFFECT FOR THIS PATIENT FOR A PERIOD > 2 WEEKS.		
4. 3/03/80:	THIS PATIENT HAS ACTIVE MEDICATIONS FOR ANTIPSYCHOTIC, ANTIDEPRESSANT, AND ANTIPARKINSON DRUGS.	8. 3/03/80:	THIS PATIENT HAS A DIAGNOSIS OF DEPRESSIVE NEUROSES AND IS RECEIVING ECT.
5. 3/03/80:	THIS PATIENT HAS INTRAMUSCULAR PSYCHOTROPIC MEDICATION WHICH HAS BEEN IN EFFECT FOR MORE THAN 10 DAYS.	9. 3/10/80:	THIS PATIENT HAS A LITHIUM BLOOD LEVEL GREATER THAN 1.5 MILLIEQUIVALENTS PER LITER.
	*(FLUPHENAZINE DECANOATE AND FLUPHENAZINE ENANTHATE WILL NOT TRIGGER THIS ALERT.)	10. 3/10/80:	THIS PATIENT IS ON LITHIUM AND NO LITHIUM LEVEL HAS BEEN REPORTED FOR MORE THAN 30 DAYS.

Figure 3. Alert statements.

tests that are already in the system that are part of this protocol, and identifies what other tests should be done (figure 5). If she orders lithium and there is a test result that is not in the file that is part of the protocol, the lithium will not be dispensed. The pharmacy will check with the physician, and the physician can authorize an override. The database then either has all the results that are part of the protocol or the clinician's override. This system was changed, and now we have our Lithium Guideline System.

In this case the physician orders the lithium and then is provided with the lithium workup sheet. We should note that even the people who create protocols follow them only 20% of the time. We have here a classic example of what the computer can do if given a chance. The follow-up system is in place. The computer

CLINICAL LABORATORY PATIENT SUMMARY REPORT

AS OF: 12/20/81

40025   MISS SMITH, BARBARA   AGE: 41   THERAPIST: FERRERO, V.   SEC. A

_____ CHEMISTRY _____

CHEMISTRY PROFILE

	FASTING-INFO	GLUC	BUN	UR-ACID	PHOS
		70-105	8-25	2.3-6.0	0.8-1.5
		MG/DL	MG/DL	MG/DL	MMOL/L
		S=3	S=1	S=0.2	S=0.07
> 12/18/81	FBS	89	19	*6.4	1.2

	CA	CHOL	PROT-T	BILI-T
	2.20-2.58	130-270	6.6-8.4	< 1.2
	MMOL/L	MG/DL	G/DL	MG/DL
	S=0.04	S=9	S=0.1	S=0.2
> 12/18/81	2.34	264	7.1	0.9

LIVER	ALK-PHOS	SGOT	SGPT	LDH
FUNCTION	25-100	5-30	5-30	100-300
	U/L	U/L	U/L	U/L
	S=3	S=2	S=2	S=12
> 12/18/81	98	21	19	156

_____ DRUG ANALYSIS _____

LITH
<1.50
MMOL/L
S=0.02

# (2)	
11/30/81	1.22
12/07/81	1.20
12/14/81	1.41
12/17/81	1.45
> 12/21/81	*1.51

ROF = RESULT ON FILE IN MED. REC.   # = MORE RESULTS ON FILE (LAST 5 PRINTED)
* = RESULTS ABNORMAL AND/OR SIGNIFICANT AND/OR NOT WITHIN THERAPEUTIC RANGE
> = NEW RESULTS   NOTE: 2 ABNORMAL OCCURRENCES INCLUDED IN NEW RESULTS

THERAPIST'S INITIALS: _____   DATE: _____ / _____ / _____

REPORT NO. 40-7CMQ-4   DISTRIBUTION: CLIN. LAB., BRD 1, MED. SERV., FERRERO, V.

Figure 4. The Institute of Living clinical laboratory patient summary report as of: 12/20/81.

THE INSTITUTE OF LIVING
HARTFORD, CONN.

BROWN,
MISS BARBARA
40028   BRD1

LITHIUM WORKUP SHEET
AS OF: 3/10/82

PAGE 1

AGE: 42   PHYSICIAN: PROCTOR, A.
PHYSICAL / NEUROLOGICAL EXAM: 1/18/82

SECTION: A
EKG: 1/26/82

_____ HEMATOLOGY _____

BLOOD CELL PROFILE	WBC 5.0-10.0	RBC 4.20-5.40	HGB 12.0-16.0 G%	HCT 36.0-47.0 %
12/31/81	5.6	4.78	14.5	42.6

INDICES	MCV 82.0-99.0	MCH 27.0-33.0	MCHC 32.0-36.0
12/31/81	87.0	29.3	33.1

	PLATE-EST
12/31/81	NORMAL

_____ NUCLEAR MEDICINE _____

T3+T4	T3-RES 31.0-45.0 %	T4 4.5-11.5 MICRO G/DL	FREE-THYROX-INDEX 4.5-11.5 MICRO G/DL
1/03/82	40.0	10.1	10.0

_____ URINALYSIS _____

URINE R + M	APPEARANCE	SPEC GRAV 1.003-1.030	HGB 0	KETONES 0	SUGAR 0 %	PROTEIN 0
12/16/81	0	1.022	0	0	0	*1+

	PH 4.8-7.8	WBC 4-5 /HPF		RBC 2-3 /HPF		CAST 0 /LPF
12/16/81	*4.0	0		0		0

_____ LITHIUM WORKUP TESTS REQUIRED _____

ELECTROLYTES, CREATININE, CBC, T3, URINE R+M

REPORT NO. 21-1CJF-1   DISTRIBUTION: PROCTOR, A.

Figure 5. The Institute of Living, Hartford, Conn. Lithium workup sheet as of: 3/10/82.

automatically generates orders at the appropriate times and provides a reminder to the physician so that she can override when the test is not required.

Recently, someone requested a list of all abnormal lithium results for a patient Smith. We provided this information from a terminal, a chronological listing of all the abnormal lithium levels. This is a "good news/bad news" situation. The good news is the request was made and the information was provided. The bad news is the physician did not use the terminal and request the information himself.

There are good reasons for this. The basic problem is that the physician must talk to the computer in computer language. This is not simple, especially if not done on a regular basis. However, there are available "tools" that solve this problem. Clout is a tool, a software product that allows retrieval from a relational database using plain English. The user builds his own vocabulary. Clout costs $400 on the microcomputer. A similar capability costs $70,000 on a mainframe, but it can be worth it. If you are making million-dollar decisions and you can have accurate, timely data, maybe you can save that $70,000.

In my example, all one has to do to get that same set of lithium results out of the microcomputer, using Clout, is to type in the original question. This is what Clout understands. This is where the technology is, and the tools are only going to get better.

In conclusion I will describe a psychiatric triage form used at the Loma Linda Hospital. It has most of the components that one would expect to find in such a report. However, there are several significant characteristics (figure 6). The document resulted from data that were entered during the interview by the physician who does not touch type. (For the 200 interviews conducted, only one patient complained that the physician typed during the interview.) This application was developed by the user. The psychiatrist, who is not a programmer, developed the triage form. He is also able to make changes. There are tables in the system, such as social history items. If there is an item that is missing, he adds the item. The system was in use one month after development of the triage report was started. This report also integrates data from other

NAME: Date of Encounter: JAN 3, 1985
  SSN: 69018730   Service Connection: SC for psychiatry (less than 50%)
  Age: 64   Sex: male   Race: white.

CHIEF COMPLAINT: Been extremely anxious x 1 yr.

HISTORY OF PRESENT ILLNESS: Pt is 10%SC for nervous condition since 1940. Pt's main
symptoms consist of obsessive-compulsive behavior and sleep onset insomnia. Pt did well on
Valium for ten yrs at Long Beach VA but was withdrawn about 7 yrs ago when he moved to Yucaipa.
Pt developed severe insomnia since then. Beginning about a yr ago, he began to develop compulsion
to count things. Pt was referred to sleep laboratory, then to psychology, and now to psychiatry. Pt also
has very sick wife with multiple chronic medical problems at home.

Family history: positive for psychiatric problems
  Alcohol and drug use is: not significant.
  Pattern of use is: not maladaptive.

CURRENT MEDICATIONS: Aspirin PRN

PAST PSYCHIATRIC HISTORY: see HPI

PAST MEDICAL HISTORY: degenerative arthritis, decreased hearing.

SOCIAL HISTORY (BRIEF):
  Marital Status: married   Living Situation: with wife and/or children
  Financial Situation: sufficient   Employment: retired
  Highest Grade Attended: 16

MENTAL STATUS EXAM:

Appearance: appropriate for situation
Observed Behavior: appropriate for circumstances
Orientation: to person, place, and time   Speech: normal
Behavior Towards Interview: appropriate, unremarkable
Memory: normal
Mood: fearful
Affect: appropriate for situation, content, and in range
Thought Processes: appropriate for situation
Thought Content: illusions
Thought Content: obsessive thoughts
Judgement: adequate for obtaining food, shelter, and clothing
  Insight: understands nature of problem
  Suicidality: has thoughts but no intentions
  Homicidality: denies any thoughts or intentions

MEDICATIONS GIVEN: Doxepin 25mg tabs, 2 tabs po qhs to be increased to 4 tabs po, #60

DISPOSITION: Mental Hygiene Clinic (LLVA)

DIAGNOSES:
Axis I: Obsessive compulsive disorder (neurosis)
Axis II: Diagnosis deferred on Axis II
Axis III: Abnormal auditory function study
Axis IV: unspecified   Axis V: fair

INTERVIEWER: M.D., Ph.D.

Figure 6. Psychiatric triage form—Loma Linda VAH list Mar. 6, 1985 14:50
page 1.

sources. Because the patient had been through the admissions process, those data were already in the computer.

There are also obvious benefits from any computerized reporting system. The report is available to others. When the patient is readmitted, there is information in the computer that can be immediately made available. Because of its structure, every piece of data that has been entered is available for a search. This application was developed using a tool called Fileman. This is a programmerless system developed by the Veterans Administration. Everyone should be aware of its capabilities. It is a MUMPS system. There are 172 VA locations that will be part of a network comprised of 300 computers, 12,000 terminals, 6,000 printers, and 600 modems. All applications are transportable, even though many different computers are used. This means that if you wanted to use that psychiatric triage application, and you have an IBM PC, you can run the application. I use Fileman on our Tandem computer system.

A psychologist in our children's clinic developed a rather complete children's clinic information system by himself, using Fileman. He had never even seen a terminal before he started. That is the power of the programmerless systems that are now available.

What makes me most excited about the potential for the VA approach is that with 172 sites, there are at least 172 staff members with a pet project, that is, something he or she really wants to do and has the expertise in. Each person can invest the time to develop an application, knowing it will go into a pool where it will be used by others if it is valuable. In turn, he or she will save time by using someone else's application that meets one of his or her needs. In this way the expertise of that whole community becomes available. This is where the technology has allowed us to go.

How can we make computer applications more successful? First, the new generation of psychiatrists are computer-ready. Second, the tools like Fileman and Clout, which allow anyone to use computers without programmers, are now available. Third, whole systems are being developed that provide data integration with management control, as exemplified by the VA system.

11

A MICROCOMPUTER-BASED MANAGEMENT INFORMATION SYSTEM FOR CONTINUING TREATMENT PSYCHIATRIC REHABILITATION PROGRAMS

Samuel Seiffer

Continuing treatment programs that serve the chronically mentally ill present unusual and at times difficult problems for systems developers in the mental health field. The patients served by continuing treatment programs tend to remain in these programs for extended periods of time, and the need to keep extensive service histories can become a burden for agencies that typically place most of their resources in direct services. Nevertheless, the bureaucratic imperatives of municipal- and state-level reporting, as well as billing and internal accountability, must be satisfied.

Before the advent of the microcomputer, attempts at computerization produced mixed results. In part this resulted from the fact that earlier systems were conceptualized and programmed to meet the needs of a wide variety of service providers, each of which had its own idiosyncratic organization, clinical approach, and informational needs. Simply put, these systems, using the lowest common denominator approach, frequently commercially developed and running on mainframe computers, could not respond to locally defined needs.

Since the development of the microcomputer in the late 1970s, and most notably since the introduction of the IBM Personal Computer in 1982, it has become possible to consider the distribution of data processing. More important, it has become economically feasible to develop highly customized applications programs to meet very localized needs. Rather than allowing the computer system to dictate clinical program design and operations, it is now possible to design computer systems around already existing programs. The discussion that follows describes the experiences of the Sound View-Throgs Neck Community Mental Health Center (SVTN-CMHC) as it automated certain key functions of its continuing treatment psychiatric rehabilitation program using a distributed microcomputer model.

THE PROBLEM

Continuing treatment programs in a free-standing community mental health center must address four major concerns. First, the program must be able to keep and have available accurate records of patient attendance. Second, the program must be able to report summary statistics for state and municipal funding sources. Third, the program must be able to generate the necessary data for medicaid and other types of billing. Finally, the program should ideally have the necessary internal data to monitor staff productivity and patient utilization of specific continuing treatment services.

Since most continuing treatment programs either directly or indirectly receive public funding, the medical record must clearly show the nature of the services provided. Typically, these services are a combination of activity, work and socialization groups. Since a patient may be in a number of such groups in the course of the day and usually has a treatment plan custom-designed for him or her, information must be collated from a large number of disparate persons and documents.

Reporting in New York State is done on the LS2c form, which categorizes continuing treatment patient visits in terms of the amount of time spent in the program in a day. For example, a patient may be in one activity group in the morning for two hours and another in the afternoon for two hours, for a total time spent in the program of four hours. By New York State regulation, this corresponds to a half-day visit.

Medicaid billing for continuing treatment programs corresponds to reporting requirements. Medicaid is therefore billed on the basis of patient time spent in the program. However, the documentation necessary to support the billing in the event of an audit must disclose the extent and nature of the services provided. This is taken to mean the specific group activities the patient participated in and the amount of time spent in these activities. In addition, a progress note must be written every two weeks. Since current practice does not allow for machine-generated progress notes, this could not be automated. At the time the SVTN medical records system was developed, a monthly rehabilitation summary form was designed to fulfill the legal requirements for documentation of continuing treatment programs. The practical problems of completing this form were addressed in extensive discussions among administrative staff at this time. Information from original attendance sheets prepared at the time activity groups are held must be transferred to a patient-specific chart. No satisfactory solution to this problem was ever arrived at, and the problem was allowed to persist. In small programs this may not be a burden. However, in a program that serves 275 different patients in the course of a month, manual completion of such a document is impractical. As systems analysis proceeded it became clearly evident that the rehabilitation summary could be properly completed only by an automated system.

One of the problems SVTN program administrators faced internally was how to gauge individual staff productivity and program utilization. Some groups would appear to be filled to capacity, although actual attendance was low. Other groups could probably be expanded to meet excess demand. Low utilization of a particular group could also be indicative of misallocated staff. Perhaps the same group run by another staff member would be more successful. Whatever the question, reliable internal utilization data in a usable form was difficult to develop manually.

SYSTEMS DEVELOPMENT

Systems development was divided into two stages. The first stage provided for an automated scheduling system for all continuing treatment patients. This scheduling subsystem would also produce the central reporting document for recording group attendance, the Group Attendance Sheet (GAS), a job previously performed manually by clerical employees. The second stage of the systems development process was to be the implementation of a computerized service recording system, which would also produce the necessary service summary for insertion into the medical record (exclusive of the biweekly progress note). Shortly after systems development began it became obvious that the implementation of a scheduling system would have to become the second stage of the system, and the service recording system would become the first application implemented. Initial discussions with program staff provided convincing evidence that line staff were unprepared to handle the paperwork demands of a scheduling system for a complex program. Scheduling for clients had, over the years, become ritualized, with an initial schedule prepared on intake. Of course, patient schedules change and in some cases quite radically. However, the written schedule for each patient was rarely revised to reflect these changes. In this instance the patient schedule after a few weeks bore little resemblance to the actual activities attended. It is significant to emphasize that problems such as the above are not data-processing problems per se but human problems of management, organization, and the overall system. They do make automated systems more difficult to implement, however.

These problems were exacerbated by an ambivalent program administration. Although the program director reacted positively to the concept of computerization and was well aware of the deficiencies of the manual system, he was unfamiliar with the systems development and implementation process. Since the director of information services had substantial familiarity with issues such as direct service staff resistance to changes in paperwork routine, problems in this area were expected. At the outset of system design and implementation, the director of information services met with the direct service staff. The responses of the staff varied from warmly positive to outright hostility. Moreover, the ambivalence of the program director was clearly in evidence and perceived accurately by his staff. A decision was made after this negative experience not to meet with program staff as a group and to confine most communication at the development level to administrative staff. Other program staff would be oriented to the system at a more appropriate time. Problems resulting from lack of experience and knowledge in this area are common to many service delivery organizations. Further, it is important to recognize that major changes of the type some envisioned can by themselves be sources of anxiety.

When systems development was commenced, a deliberate decision was made to produce an automated system that would look and function as much like the preexisting system as possible, except that the informational flow would now be accelerated. Many of the frontline service delivery staff had experienced several other automated systems used by SVTN over the years. None of these systems had addressed the core needs of the agency and were therefore quite reasonably seen as a burden with no visible payoff.

Group attendance data are gathered on the Group Attendance Sheet (GAS), which, in addition to stub information regarding date and staff members present for the group, lists the names and case numbers of the patients scheduled for the group and whether they are absent or present. This sheet is retained, except that some further information is now requested (see figure 1). A similar sheet, the Daily Activity Sheet (DAS) is used to record individual patient contacts.

The concept of the rehabilitation services MIS system (RSMIS) is that processing, including initial data entry, would be performed locally, with outputs generated locally and, where appropriate, given either to the medical records office, in the case of rehabilitation summaries, or to the central MIS office, as in the case of the Daily Visit Report. Managerial reports programmed at the request of the unit director would be locally generated and retained at the unit

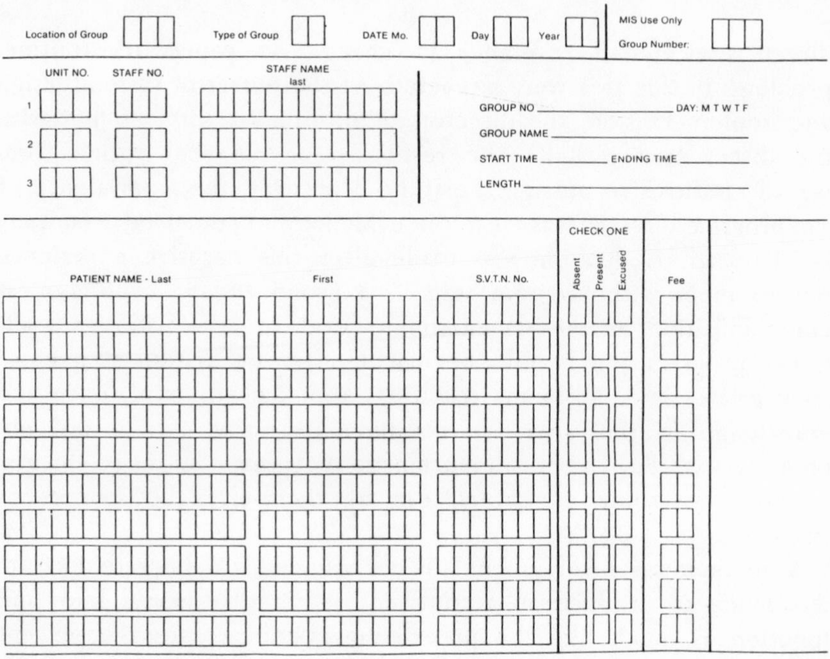
Location of Group
Type of Group
DATE Mo.
Day
Year
MIS Use Only
Group Number:
UNIT NO.
STAFF NO.
STAFF NAME
last
1
2
3
GROUP NO
DAY: M T W T F
GROUP NAME
START TIME
ENDING TIME
LENGTH
CHECK ONE
PATIENT NAME - Last
First
S.V.T.N. No.
Absent
Present
Excused
Fee

Figure 1. Group Attendance Sheet.

level. Since copies of all data are retained in the central MIS office, productivity data can always be supplied to the executive director and associate director as requested.

Since SVTN's computers are not networked, the system as designed would have to function autonomously at the machine level. However, at the systems level the rehabilitation services MIS system was deliberately conceived as being a part of a larger clinic-wide management information system. It was hoped that by conceptualizing the rehabilitation system as part of a larger system, the problems of system fragmentation and Balkanization could be avoided, even though staff operating the system at the unit level were not directly responsible to the director of information services. Figure 2 shows schematically the organization and paperwork flow arrived at for the rehabilitation services MIS system.

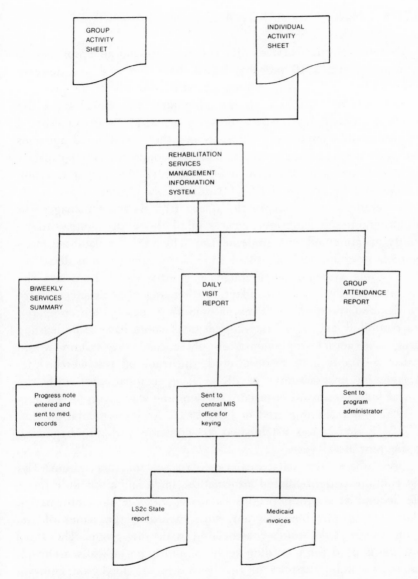

Figure 2. Paperwork flow and organization of the Rehabilitation Services Management Information System.

PROGRAMMING AND HARDWARE

The rehabilitation services MIS system is run on an Epson Equity I computer with a 10 megabyte hard disk drive and one diskette drive. Unfortunately, the choice of hardware was made prior to systems development, due to the long lead time needed for the necessary municipal purchase approval process. This was exacerbated by questionable purchasing practices in other city-funded agencies that were unrelated in any way to SVTN. A somewhat larger-capacity machine would probably have been desirable. The output function is supported by an Epson FX-100 dot matrix printer.

Programming was done in the dBase III+ database management and programming language. This enabled the entire system to be rapidly programmed and implemented. The use of a database management program such as dBase III+ has advantages and disadvantages. While systems development is greatly speeded up and the system is relatively easy to adapt to changing circumstances, there is a decided trade-off in terms of operating speed when compared to a compiled language. Since a great deal would have to be learned during the actual implementation phase, and the system would almost inevitably have to be altered, the trade-off was worthwhile. Further, by programming in dBase III+, compatibility with the central MIS system was ensured. Programming was begun in February of 1987 and was completed in June 1987. An implementation date of July 1, 1987, was established, to coincide with the beginning of the new fiscal year.

Three dBase III+ databases were created for this system. The first contains patient-related information, including a schedule form. The second is a group profile database and contains information related to groups the program runs, including the name of the group and a code number associated with the group. The third database is used for recording services, and is periodically archived, due to the finite capacity of the hard disk on the Epson Equity I computer.

Menu programs were generated by the program generator supplied with the dBase III+ program. The output from this program generator needed substantial modification to work conveniently for operational staff. In fact, the menu programs were customized to meet the work habits acquired in former jobs. The ability to customize the menu system created a very positive response in this area. Input and report programs were written from scratch, because they needed more complex routines and output formats than could be automatically generated. The screen "painting" utility of dBase III+ was useful in giving the input screens a well-organized and neat appearance. It also helped speed up the screen layout process somewhat by cutting down on the amount of trial-and-error coding that is necessary for complex systems.

OPERATIONS

The most difficult aspect of systems implementation is not the technical problem of systems analysis or programming, but the human problem of orienting staff to an automated system. Two groups of staff had to be trained and oriented immediately: those staff delivering direct services to patients, and the staff who actually had the day-to-day responsibility for inputting data and generating reports. At the time, the rehabilitation service had as a clerical employee a person who had worked for some years in a commercial data processing operation. In this case, skills learned in the commercial world were easily transferred to the clinic setting, although this person experienced some difficulty in getting used to the microcomputer, having been trained on a minicomputer system. An unanticipated problem was experienced in implementing a back-up system for the computer operator's job. In the manual system the backup was unsystematic, simply because the job involved no technical training, and the manual transcription process required only rudimentary clerical skills. Moreover, since the paperwork was already running far behind schedule, an absence on the part of the person who was regularly assigned to prepare the Daily Visit Report and the Monthly Rehabilitation Summary simply meant that the work would be done one or more days late.

A computerized system creates needs and a momentum of its own. Work cannot be held over, or the job of catching up becomes increasingly difficult. Therefore, considerable effort was put into training back-up personnel within the rehabilitation unit clerical pool. In this case it was necessary to train several persons who lacked any knowledge at all of computers and data entry tasks.

Because the system was designed to be as transparent as possible for direct service staff, forms and procedures were familiar. However, some problems emerged. In the manual system to be abandoned a good deal of sloppiness could be tolerated in paperwork. For example, patient case numbers were frequently absent from clinician report sheets. Since these numbers were not needed for data input, the requirement that clinician reporting sheets (GAS and individual sheets) arrive at the unit office complete and legible met with some resistance. This was mitigated somewhat by the knowledge on the part of direct service staff that by omitting information they were only making the job of the unit clerk more difficult. A second problem arose when both administrative and line staff made ad hoc changes in the clinical program or in the times of already existing groups without letting either the director of information services or data entry personnel know. Fortunately the system itself was designed to be sufficiently robust to respond to this lapse. However, lack of sensitivity and awareness of the needs of an automated system remains a problem.

SYSTEM OUTPUTS

To date there are three major system outputs.

1. *The Daily Visit Report.* (See figure 3.) The program for this report selects the patient contacts for a specified day, sums the total patient time spent in the program for the day and prints out a computation of the type of visit to be reported to the state and billed to medicaid if applicable. The information on this report is keyed into the central MIS system to accomplish these tasks. It is anticipated that eventually the Daily Visit Report will be output simultaneously to both diskettes, and the hard copy will serve as a backup for audit purposes. By outputting this report to disk and having the central MIS computer input via magnetic media, considerable keying time will be saved.

DAILY VISIT REPORT

			FD	HD	B		
				VISIT			
GOLD	DAVID	1431901	X				7.00
MARTIN	ANDREW	1431951			X		1.00
RILEY	RICHARD	1432021			X		2.00
O'CONNOR	MICHAEL	1432271			X		2.50
FOLEY	DORIS	1432321		X			4.84
WILLIAMS	BEATRICE	1432431	X				5.00
RUSSO	ANTHONY	1432491	X				5.50
PETERS	PEARL	1432621			X		2.00
ANSER	ADELE	1440021			X		2.00
VITALE	VIRGINIA	1440121		X			3.00
KINGMAN	ELAINE	1440131			X		2.00
REGAN	LUIS	1440141			X		1.50
GATES	WILLIAM	1440201			X		2.00
GALLUP	BENJAMIN	1440591			X		1.50
KEYES	JOSEPH	1440621			X		2.00
REZNICK	RUTH	1440681			X		2.00
DOWD	DOUGLAS	1440801			X		2.00
ELLEN	JOSEPH	1441431			X		2.00
BROOKINGS	EDDIE	1441511		X			3.50
WHITE	THOMAS	1442231			X		2.84
MATHEWS	MIRIAM	1442261			X		2.00
RIVERA	RITA	1450001			X		2.00
ARNOLD	DENNIS	1450031		X			4.50
WREN	CHRISTOPHER	2419981	X				5.00
DESALVO	DOLORES	2432471		X			4.34

Figure 3. Daily Visit Report.

2. *The Biweekly Rehabilitation Summary.* (See figure 4.) The program for this report selects the patient contacts for a specified two-week period and, by accessing the group profile database, prints out a descriptive listing of patient services received during the specified period. There is a preprinted space on the output form for the required biweekly progress note. After the note has been written this summary and note become part of the patient's permanent medical record.

3. *The Attendance Report.* This report provides a numerical count of the attendance in each group conducted on any specified day. It is intended to give the program director a clear idea of how the clinical program is being utilized.

RESULTS

The rehabilitation services MIS system has now been in operation for two years. As a result of this system a major backlog of paperwork has been cleared. More important, this backlog has not reappeared. Further, a large amount of staff time which would have gone into clerical work is now available for other necessary tasks. Most important, total compliance with medicaid record-keeping requirements has been achieved. The data in the patient record will always agree with the billing because the information source for billing and the case record is the same. This type of integration between component parts of the total system is important and, unfortunately, sometimes overlooked.

Because unit line staff were able to see an observable payoff in the form of easier and more timely record keeping as well as a decreased overall clerical workload, the system has legitimated and institutionalized itself. That some staff were unhappy with more stringent paperwork requirements was expected and understandable. Bad habits die hard.

At the time the RSMIS system was being designed and implemented, the work experience component of the rehabilitation pro-

BIWEEKLY REHABILITATION SUMMARY

Name of patient	SVTN #	From	To
	1410291	11/01/87	11/15/87

SUMMARY OF REHABILITATION SERVICES

DATE	NAME OF GROUP	STAFF IN GROUP			UNIT	TIME OF GROUP	DURATION
11/02/87	Bldg Main PM	0819			303	12:30-03:00	2.50
11/02/87	Ind Counsel.	0733			303	—	0.50
11/03/87	Workshop PM1	0819			303	12:30-03:00	2.50
11/03/87	Therapy	0867	0712		303	09:00-10:00	1.00
11/04/87	Bldg Main PM	0819			303	12:30-03:00	2.50
11/05/87	Bldg Main PM	0819			303	12:30-03:00	2.50
11/06/87	Voc. Therapy	0371	0711	0733	303	01:00-02:00	1.00
11/09/87	Bldg Main PM	0819			303	12:30-03:00	2.50
11/10/87	Bldg Main PM	0819			303	12:30-03:00	2.50
11/10/87	Therapy	0867			303	09:00-10:00	1.00
11/11/87	Bldg Main PM	0819	0711		303	12:30-03:00	2.50
11/12/87	Bldg Main PM	0819			303	12:30-03:00	2.50
11/13/87	Bldg Main AM	0819			303	08:30-11:30	3.00
11/13/87	Voc. Therapy	0371	0711	0733	303	01:00-02:00	1.00
11/13/87	Ind Counsel.	0733			303	—	0.50

Summary note for: 11/01/87 to 11/15/87

Sig. of rehab. coordinator	Date	Sig. of treat. coordinator	Date

ROBERT   WRIGHT   0733   ROBERT   COLE   0733

Figure 4. Biweekly Rehabilitation Services Summary.

gram was being greatly expanded. This presented some major problems for the system. The original concept of the scheduling system that allowed for 25 time blocks for the week was inadequate. The service recording system continues to function well. When the scheduling component of the RSMIS system is implemented, some thought may have to be given to redesign in order to accommodate a program that does not fit into the normal working day.

Has the RSMIS system had any programmatic impact in terms of the data's utilization as an evaluation tool? It is probably much too early to assess this accurately. Large, complex mental health programs are not quickly or easily reshaped. Moreover the manifest function of the RSMIS was not to directly reshape programs—this is properly the province of administrators directly responsible for the program. The data the RSMIS system gathers do not aim at program review. What is clear, if only by impression and inference, is a developing consciousness that data are being gathered and feedback is being communicated to concerned administrators. By this means the rehabilitation services MIS system has had the latent function of making staff aware of their responsibilities to the clinic and to the continuing treatment program. It may well be that the most important contribution of the rehabilitation services MIS system has is to create the structure and conditions under which more sophisticated program-oriented reviews can take place in the future.

PART V

COMPUTER UTILIZATION IN COMMUNITY MENTAL HEALTH CENTERS

12

A NATIONWIDE SURVEY OF COMPUTER UTILIZATION IN COMMUNITY MENTAL HEALTH CENTERS

David Baskin
and Samuel Seiffer

High technology and computers have been rapidly making their way into health care systems and in particular into the mental health service delivery system. To date, no examination on a nationwide basis has been made as to how computers are being used in mental health. This study examines this issue.

It is an interesting coincidence that the first initial staffing grants for community mental health centers (CMHCs) were made at about the same time that large mainframe computers became available to the medical, educational and business worlds. Most CMHCs, in spite of much encouragement and some early pioneering experimentation, were unable to take advantage of the computer until the 1970s, when minicomputers became available. Throughout the 1970s a steady stream of publications emanated from National Institute of Mental Health, encouraging CMHCs to develop systematic, computerized management information systems. Still, the technology of data processing was largely unavailable to many, if not most, small-

and medium-sized centers. The minicomputers then available required relatively highly trained personnel to write software and operate the systems.

The advent of the low-cost microcomputer has once again spurred efforts at automating the informational needs of CMHCs. Although the first microcomputers were introduced in 1976, it was several years more before microcomputers useful for medical, commercial, and educational applications became available, along with easily usable software. As CMHCs entered the 1980s, computer technology advanced dramatically. Microcomputer memory size increased and, perhaps more important, data storage devices capable of handling large databases became available. Further, competitive forces within the computer industry have brought computers within the reach of most mental health centers.

Given the immense impact of these recent advances in computer technology, it is now appropriate to determine how these developments have affected CMHCs nationwide. The purpose of this chapter is to report the result of a nationwide survey of community mental health centers' utilization of computers.

REVIEW OF THE LITERATURE

Although computers have been commercially available since the 1960s, it is only recently that they have become accessible to large numbers of noncomputer professionals in the mental health field. Because of this there has been little systematic investigation of their use. The most wide-ranging work regarding the development of diverse mental health applications for computers was done by Laska and Bank (1975). Their work on the Multi-State Management Information System (MSIS) focused on the development of regional and state reporting mechanisms. More recently, Baer, Gastfriend, and Rosenbaum (1984) have addressed the problems of establishing a microcomputer database for outpatient psychopharmacology. A number of writers, among them Hammer, Lyons, and Strain (1985) and Booker and Platman (1985) have described varying approaches to total decentralized microcomputer systems in psychiatry.

Meier and Geiger (1985) recently conducted a limited survey of current or expected use of computers in a mental health setting. Their software survey revealed that most respondents made very little use of a host of functions but that they expected to make more use in the future. Of the uses currently utilized, many of the traditional uses of computers in their field emerged prominently: clerical, data analyses, evaluation, and administration. The approach of those responsible for operating the mental health system seems to be oriented toward mechanizing those functions already identified as essential to the operation of the service delivery system. The balance of the literature in the field is composed mainly of self-help articles, such as that by Greist (1983), devoted to selecting a computer system for a mental health center, or the application of specific discussions, such as one by Schwartz, Stinson, and Berlant (1985), which deals with clinical uses of computers, dedicating only slight attention to the wide variety of alternative uses.

METHOD

A total of 648 community mental health centers were sent questionnaires requesting information in regard to characteristics of their respective centers and of their utilization of computers. Two hundred and fifty-six (256) centers responded, constituting a 40% response rate. Of the individuals who responded to the questionnaire, 34% were directors or associate directors, 16% were administrators, 9% were data information system processing managers, and the remaining 41% had some other job title.

The areas covered in the questionnaire were as follows:

I. Characteristics of the center
   A. Center location
   B. NIMH region
   C. Yearly outpatient admissions
   D. Yearly outpatient visits
   E. Number of clinical/nonclinical staff

II. Characteristics of MIS
   A. Manual or computer system
   B. Year in which MIS was established
   C. Functions of the MIS

III. Computerization facets
   A. Type of computer used
   B. Experience with service bureaus
   C. Whether CMHC is part of larger data processing system
   D. How data is processed (interactive vs. batch)
   E. Type of peripherals
   F. Storage/memory capacities of computer
   G. Types of software/packages used
   H. Personnel and costs of system

IV. Assessment of systems
   A. Cost & efficiency evaluations
   B. Current system vis-à-vis service bureau

Percentages cited may not always total 100%, due to rounding differences.

The distribution of center locations were as follows:

Center location	Number	Percentage
City (population> 500,000)	42	(17)
Small city/town	182	(73)
Village	20	(8)
Suburb of a city	4	(2)

The center locations were distributed among the 10 NIMH regions as follows:

	I	II	III	IV	V	VI	VII	VIII	IX	X
Number =	28	23	23	64	36	15	13	17	14	12

Total: 245
Missing data:11

The number of yearly outpatient admissions were are follows:

Admissions	Number	Percentage
1-999	52	(21)
1,000-1,499	55	(22)
1,500-2,499	69	(28)
2,500 +	69	(28)

The number of yearly outpatient visits were as follows:

Yearly visits	Number	Percentage
<13,000	60	(25)
13,001-20,000	55	(23)
20,001-40,000	63	(27)
>40,000	60	(25)

The number of clinical staff was as follows:

Number of clinical staff	Number	Percentage
<30	54	(24)
30-44	56	(25)
45-70	59	(26)
>70	58	(26)

The number of nonclinical (support) staff was as follows:

Number of nonclinical staff	Number	Percentage
≤14	54	(24)
15-22	55	(25)
23-42	59	(27)
43≤	55	(25)

RESULTS

Management Information System

With regard to management information systems (MIS), 61 centers report having manual systems; 220 indicate that their systems are computerized; and eight centers state that they have no MIS. Of those that have an MIS, 39 (18%) established one between 1955 and 1974; 60 (28%) commenced operations between 1975 and 1977; 45 (21%) began between 1978 and 1979; and 68 (32%) established an MIS between 1980 and 1984 (see Table 1). NIMH Region 2 (New York, New Jersey, Puerto Rico, and the Virgin Islands) seems to have been the last region to have developed an MIS. The functions handled by MIS were as follows:

Function	N
Caseload	229
Client visit data	233
Billing	204
Budget and accounting	176
Staff productivity	225
Inventory	73
Payroll	148
Research and evaluation	253
Other miscellaneous uses	46

Computerization

Of those centers that have computerized, only 52 (24%) did so prior to 1977; 40 (19%) computerized from 1978 to 1979; 58 (27%) did so between 1980 and 1981; and 65 (30%) computerized from 1982 to 1984 (see Table 2). NIMH Regions 2 and 5 seem to have been the last to computerize.

The types of computers used were as follows: 60 (27%) had in-

Table 1. Year MIS System Established by NIMH Region

		1	2	3	4	5	6	7	8	9	10	Row Total
1974 or Earlier	N	4	4	6	9	6	2	2	2	2	2	39
	%	(15)	(31)	(30)	(16)	(17)	(17)	(18)	(12)	(17)	(18)	
1975–1979	N	15	2	9	31	15	5	7	10	7	4	105
	%	(58)	(15)	(45)	(56)	(43)	(42)	(64)	(59)	(58)	(36)	
1980 or Later	N	7	7	5	15	14	5	2	5	3	5	68
	%	(27)	(54)	(25)	(27)	(40)	(42)	(18)	(29)	(25)	(46)	
Column Total		26	13	20	55	35	12	11	17	12	11	212

Table 2. Year of Computerization by NIMH Region

		1	2	3	4	5	6	7	8	9	10	Row Total
1974 or Earlier	N %			3 (18)	4 (7)	1 (3)		1 (10)	1 (6)	1 (8)		11
1975–1979	N %	12 (48)	2 (15)	6 (35)	19 (32)	13 (34)	6 (50)	6 (60)	6 (35)	5 (42)	6 (50)	81
1980 or Later	N %	13 (52)	11 (85)	8 (47)	36 (61)	24 (63)	6 (50)	3 (30)	10 (59)	6 (50)	6 (50)	123
Column Total		25	13	17	59	38	12	10	17	12	12	215

house microcomputers; 75 (34%) had in-house minicomputers; 29 (13%) had in-house mainframes; 53 (24%) used outside mainframes and 2 had outside mini- or microcomputers; 40 centers had a combination of different types (micro-, mini- or mainframe) of computers. A total of 159 (78%) centers report that they own their computers, 35 (17%) lease or rent computers and 10 (5%) both own and lease computers.

Only 33% of the centers indicate that they currently use a computer service bureau, but 53% say that they have used a service bureau in the past. Of those who have used a service bureau and who have experience with their own system, an overwhelming 86% indicate that in-house processing is superior, 9% report no difference in performance and only 5% deem the service bureau to be better.

Many community mental health centers are part of larger hospital systems or mental health networks such as county or state. A plurality (66%) of CMHCs likewise report that their data processing systems are part of larger processing systems. Of those having computerized systems, 64% use remote batch processing, whereas 30% have on-line systems (6% were missing data).

Regarding the brand of computer (hardware) used, IBM (35%), Digital (16%) and Texas Instruments (14%) were the most widely selected; IBM (28%) and Texas Instruments (19%) were also the most widely used peripherals, although it was not unusual to find respondents describing systems with more than one manufacturer of peripherals. Concerning the main memory and storage capacities of 64 kilobytes or less, 24% had main memory capacity between 65k and 192k; 23% had main memory capacity between 200k–320k; and 26% had main memory capacity greater than 320k. A total of 27% had mass storage capacity of 20 megabytes or less, 45% had between 22 and 96 megabytes and 28% had mass storage greater than 96m. These very crude measures of system size must be used advisedly. Merely having more available random access memory does not necessarily make for a more powerful or flexible system. Software efficiency and overall system configuration must also be considered. Nonetheless, traditional measures of system size and power do indicate the variety of system capacities now used in mental health applications.

Regarding the software utilized, 142 use custom-designed applications, 76 use some packaged applications, 58 use proprietory software specific for medical or mental health applications, 75 use database management programs, 81 use word processing programs and 24 use general application packages (such as Lotus 1-2-3). It is interesting to note that 44% of the respondents feel that at least one of their programs or packages has performed particularly well, while 23% have used programs which they have found disappointing. The majority (61%) of centers have written at least some of their own programs; the most popular programming languages used were BASIC, COBOL, and RPGII. The large number of users who have programmed applications in BASIC may be indicative of the home-grown character of much current work in mental health, since BASIC is not only rarely used in commercial programming but is regarded as cumbersome and inefficient. Those users who have programmed in COBOL or RPGII may reflect a subpopulation who have invested the time, effort, and money in higher level software development.

Concerning staffing and costs of computer systems, an average of 3.3 data processing staff were utilized. The average staffing cost was $42,384. The average capital cost was $41,931 and the average cost for expendables was $10,988. The mean percentage of center budget spent on data processing operations was 3.1%.

With regard to the perceived effect of computerization on operating costs, 40% believed that it reduced costs, 33% believed that it increased costs, and 27% believed that it had no effect. Most important, 86% contended that the computerization had increased efficiency of the organization, only 5% believed that it decreased efficiency, and 9% felt it had no effect.

It should be noted that center size (based on outpatient department admissions) was not correlated with the general type of computer (micro-, mini-, or mainframe) used.

DISCUSSION

As in all studies one must ask how generalizable the sample was in this particular study. The variability in the various center characteristics suggests that our sample was fairly representative of community mental health centers in general. Of course it is possible that only centers with more developed computer systems or more comprehensive administration responded to the survey questionnaires.

It was of interest to learn that there are still centers with no management information systems. With cuts in funding it is possible that centers have had to do without this important function. However, it is difficult to understand how centers can compute levels of service and billing without an MIS, but it is possible that some centers do not perform these functions.

Region 2, which consists of New York, New Jersey, Puerto Rico, and the Virgin Islands, surprisingly lagged in the establishment of an MIS and computerization. This was surprising in light of the fact that New York and New Jersey are often regarded as being in the forefront of new enterprises. These lags may be due to the fact that many CMHCs are part of larger institutions that limit CMHC flexibility and initiative, or the lag may be artifactual.

An important finding of the study was that even though computerization was not perceived to have reduced costs, it was perceived to increase the efficiency of the organization. This may be due to the newly recognized flexibility of microcomputers. The microcomputer, by virtue of its availability, encourages experimentation and allows management to do its own programming and to have increased control over the various data based functions. This explanation may also explain why respondents preferred their own computer systems to those of service bureaus.

Of course computerization is still an ongoing process and the variety of its functions that centers choose to computerize may increase with time. Hence it would be interesting to replicate this type of study at a later date, in view of the rapid advances in computer technology and its decreasing cost.

It should be noted that each center's categorization of micro- versus mini- versus mainframe computer systems was at times subjective. In all, users do not seem to be in agreement as to the differences between various systems. For example, several IBM System 34 (minicomputer) users described their systems as mainframes.

The significance of this study is that it has chronicled the advent of widespread utilization of computers in community mental health centers. Although this development is only recent, further studies are necessary to determine the impact of computers on the service delivery systems.

If the research to date reveals anything, it is that computers have not fundamentally altered the type of information used and accumulated. Rather, computers have altered only the form in which this information is gathered, stored, and accessed. Nonetheless, this may change in the future.

REFERENCES

Baer, L., D. Gastfriend, and G. Rosenbaum. 1984. Hardware considerations in an integrated/ research data base in psychopharmacology. *Computers in Psychiatry/Psychology* 6(3): 9–12.

Booker, T. C., and S. R. Plotman. 1985. A decentralized mental health reporting system. *Hospital and Community Psychiatry* 36(1): 2 19–21.

Greist, J. 1983. Selecting a computer system for a mental health center. *Hospital and Community Psychiatry* 34(10): 909–910.

Hammer, J., J. Lyons, and J. Strain. 1985. Evolution of a stand-alone integrated micro-computer software system for psychiatric services. *Computers in Psychiatry/Psychology* 7(1): 7–9.

Laska, E., and G. Bank. 1975. *Safeguarding psychiatric privacy: computer systems and their uses.* New York: John Wiley and Sons, 1975.

Meier, S. T., and S. Geiger. 1985. Survey of computer use in counseling centers. *Computers in Psychiatry/Psychology* 7(1): 13.

Schwartz, S. R., C. Stinson, and J. Berlant. 1985. Computers in Psychiatry. *Computers in Medical Practice* 2(2): 42–50.

NAME INDEX

SUBJECT INDEX